CW01651014

SEXUAL EDUCATION WITH QUESTIONS AND ANSWERS

SEXUAL EDUCATION

WITH QUESTIONS AND ANSWERS

Deborah P. Matthews

INVADER

FOREWORD

Adolescence is a time of change, both mentally and physically. Over several years a child's body changes visibly and the mind develops so that by the mid teens he or she is beginning to think and look more like an adult.

Although it may be a confusing time, adolescence is also exciting and it is not surprising that teenagers want to know all about the changes that they are going through. Nowadays, most subjects can be discussed openly, yet it is still sometimes difficult or embarrassing for parents to answer all their children's questions in the way they would like.

This book has been specially written to cope with those awkward or complicated questions which adolescents ask about puberty and sex.

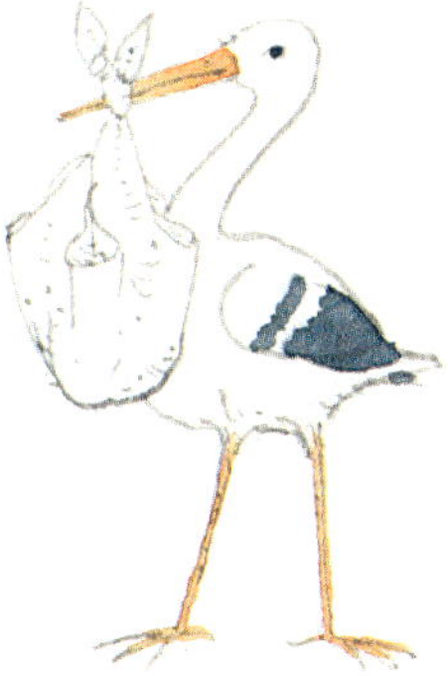

CONTENTS

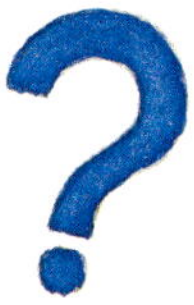

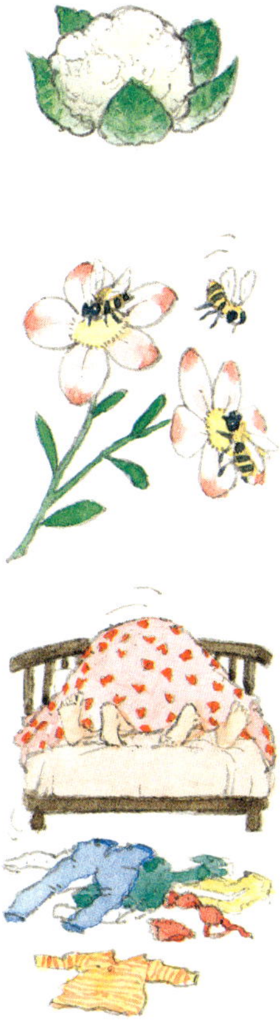
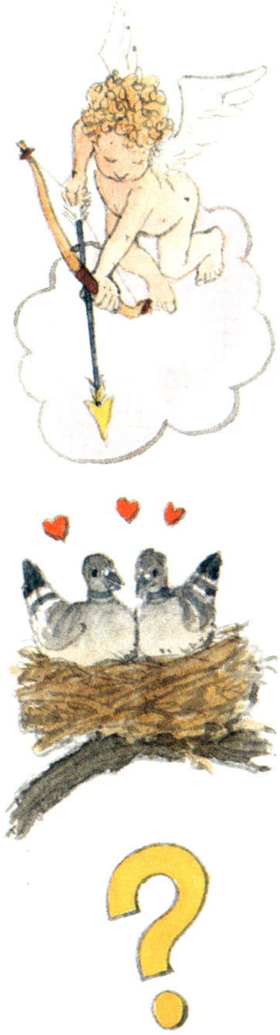
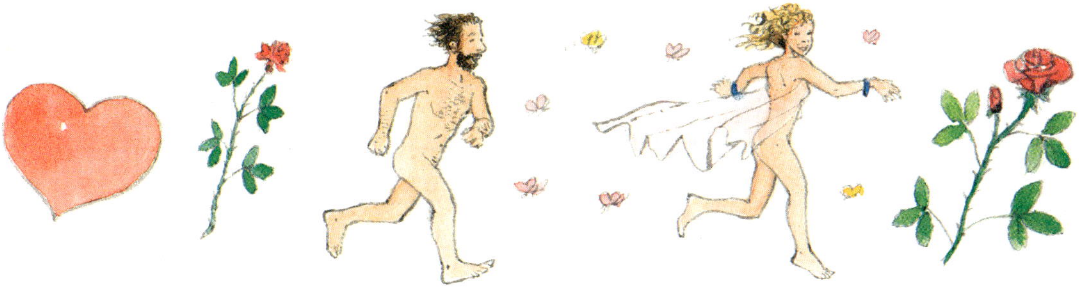

IN WHAT WAYS ARE BOYS AND GIRLS DIFFERENT?

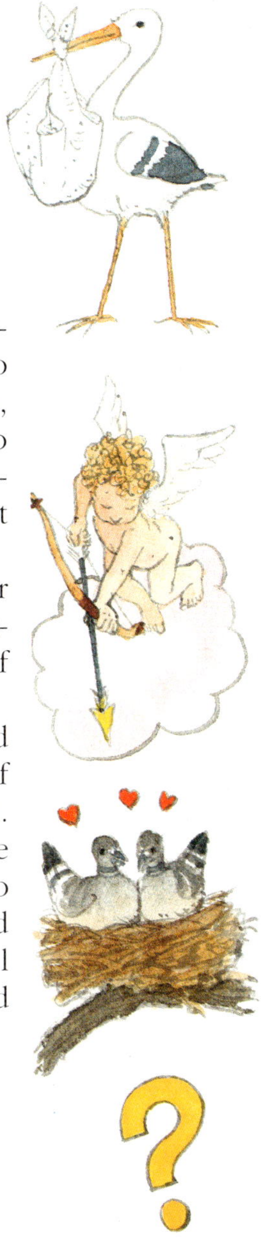

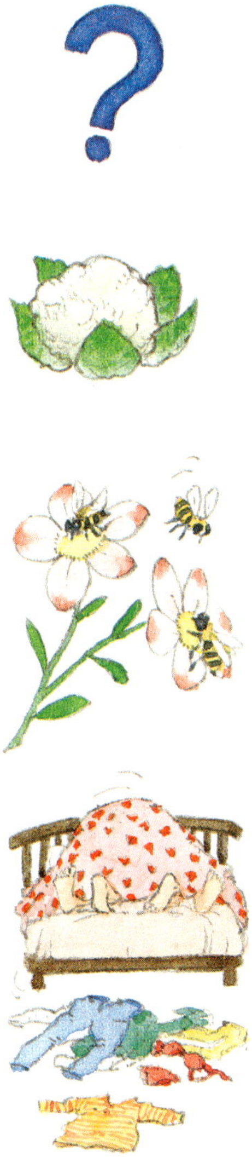

Boys and girls are very aware of certain differences between them. Boys, for example, tend to think of a typical girl as being romantic, vain, unadventurous, too well-behaved and quick to fall in love. Girls, on the other hand, see a typical boy as being tougher, uncaring, lazy about housework and too aggressive.

Are boys and girls born with these differences or does it depend on their background and upbringing? Experts think that it is a combination of hereditary genes and 'conditioning'.

In recent years, however, parents try to avoid conditioning their children because the role of the man and woman in society has changed. Women are no longer expected to stay at home all day and many fathers help their partners to look after the children and do the household chores. Nevertheless, there are fundamental differences between men and women, boys and girls, the most obvious of which is physical.

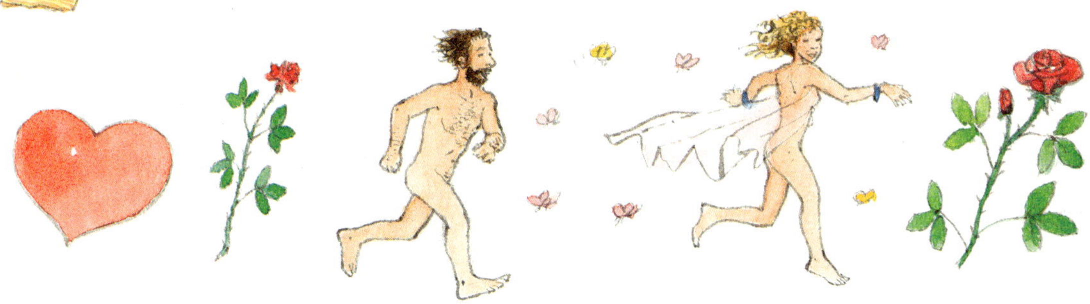

• What are the external male sexual organs?

A man's external sexual organs are the penis and the scrotum – a bag of skin which holds the testicles, or testes. The diagram below shows the different male external sexual organs.
The end of the penis is called the glans and this is protected by a loose fold of skin called the foreskin. In the middle of the glans is a small hole which is the opening for a passage called the urethra. The urethra allows either urine or semen to pass through the penis.
The scrotum holds the testicles away from the body because they function better in temperatures that are lower than body temperature.
Doctors will sometimes check that the testicles have descended properly into the scrotum. Testicles that have not descended enough will not produce sperm that are capable of fertilisation, but this can be corrected by a minor surgical operation.

The male sexual organs

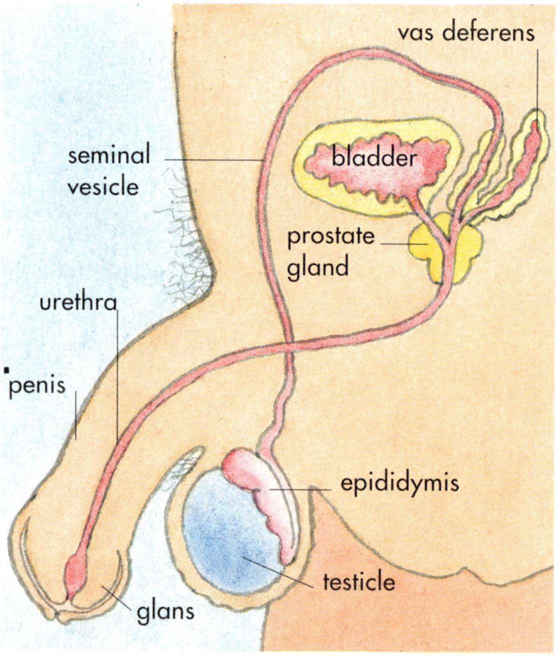

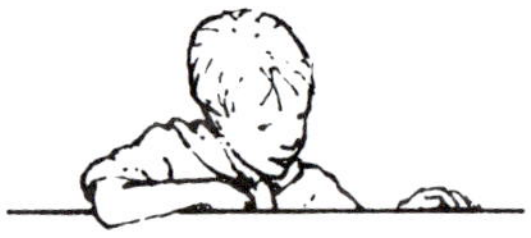

A few months ago I stopped taking showers with the boys after a football game. I was ashamed to show my penis in the showers.
It isn't very big and I thought the other boys would laugh at me.
Then, last weekend, my uncle invited me to go fishing with him. I get on really well with him and while we were out I told him all about my problem. He explained that penises grew to be all sizes and that it was better to have a small penis than one that was so big it was uncomfortable.
So after the next game I decided to join my friends in the showers. No one said anything about my penis and I remembered what my uncle had said: he was right.

Martin, 15 years old

• What are the internal male sexual organs?

The internal male sexual organs consist of two testicles, the vas deferens, the seminal vesicles and the prostate gland.
The testicles are each about the size of a large marble. The left testicle hangs slightly lower than the right one. Each testicle has many sperm ducts leading

out of it. These ducts lead into a baggy tube, called the epididymis, and this becomes a narrow tube called the vas deferens. Each vas deferens leads to a seminal vesicle and the prostate gland. The prostate gland is a sac, about the size of a horse-chestnut, which lies just below the bladder. The seminal vesicles and the bladder are connected to the urethra. Look at the diagram to see the positions of the internal sexual organs of a man.

• What are the external female sexual organs?

A woman's external sexual organs are found between a slit formed by two folds of fat. This is called the vulva. Above the vulva is the pubis which is an area of fatty tissue covering the pubic bone.

The folds of the vulva protect the labia, the clitoris, the opening of the urethra and the entrance of the vagina. The diagram clearly illustrates the two separate openings. The labia are a pair of fleshy, petal-like folds and the clitoris is a small, sensitive organ.

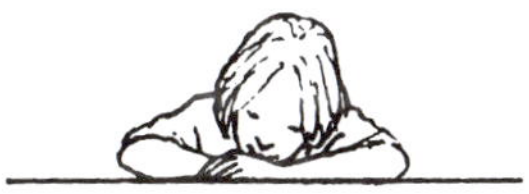

I remember when I was little and my mother was bathing my baby nephew. I was surprised when I saw his willy and I asked my mother: 'What has he got between his legs? Why haven't I got one? Did it fall off?'

Elizabeth, 11 years old

• What are the internal female sexual organs?

The internal sexual organs of a woman are the vagina, the cervix, the uterus, or womb, the Fallopian tubes, or oviducts, and the ovaries.

The vagina is a passage leading from the vulva to the cervix at the base of the uterus. This passage is capable of expanding and contracting. During childbirth it expands so that the baby can pass out.

The uterus is a pear-shaped organ about the size of a hen's egg. During pregnancy, the uterus increases in size as the baby grows.

The two Fallopian tubes lead out of the top of the uterus – one on either side. At the end of each tube is an ovary.

The ovaries are about the size of almonds.

The female sexual organs

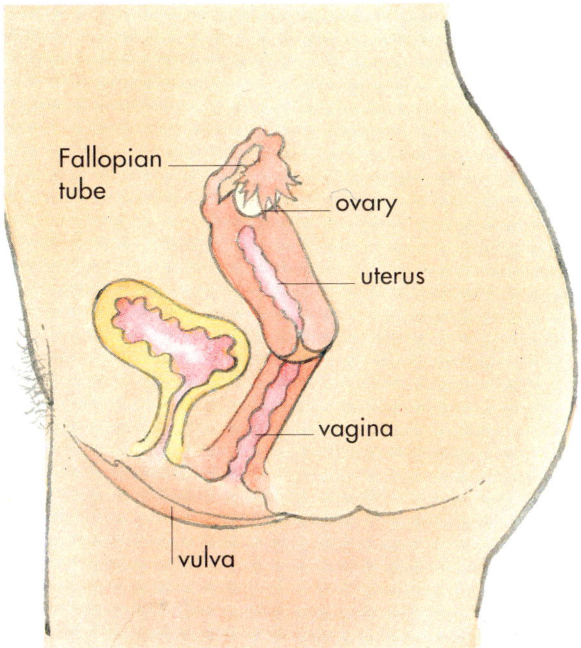

Are women 'the weaker sex'?

Men are usually physically stronger than women. This is clearly seen in sporting events. The reason for this physical difference is because in a partnership where it is the role of one person to become pregnant and bear children, the other person has to find food and defend the family territory. However, although women are generally physically weaker than men, the act of childbearing is an extraordinary physical feat in itself and the woman's role in keeping the human species alive is very important.

• What are reproductive cells, or gametes?

An amoeba is a unicellular creature. This means it consists of a single cell. In the middle of the cell is a nucleus. The nucleus controls the cell and its function. All living things, whether they are vegetables, animals or human beings, are made up of one or more cells. A human body is made up of several millions of cells.
Most of the cells are so small that they cannot be seen even under a magnifying glass, but each cell has a particular function in the whole organism. Certain cells, for example, produce the gastric juices necessary for digestion, while others, such as nerve cells, are capable of sending messages to the brain and other parts of the body.
The task of reproductive cells, or gametes, is to ensure reproduction.
The reproductive cell of the man is the sperm. The reproductive cell of the woman is the egg (the biological term for this is ovum, plural: ova). The egg is about the size of the blunt end of a needle, but the sperm is much smaller – it is invisible to the human eye.
When a sperm and an egg meet, the sperm enters the egg and the fertilised egg becomes an embryo.
However, this process is far more complex than it seems because it depends on other factors, such as hormones.

• What is a hormone?

The parts of the human body which make and secrete chemical substances are called glands.
The chemical substances they produce are known as hormones and these are secreted into the bloodstream.
As the hormones pass around the body they carry instructions to different tissues. Some hormones are responsible for making muscle cells, for example, while others ensure growth. Certain hormones trigger the production of the reproductive cells, the eggs (ova) and the sperm.
Testosterone is the male reproductive hormone. Testosterone is also produced in women, but in lesser quantities.
Oestrogen and progesterone are the female reproductive hormones and they are also to be found in minute quantities in the male body.

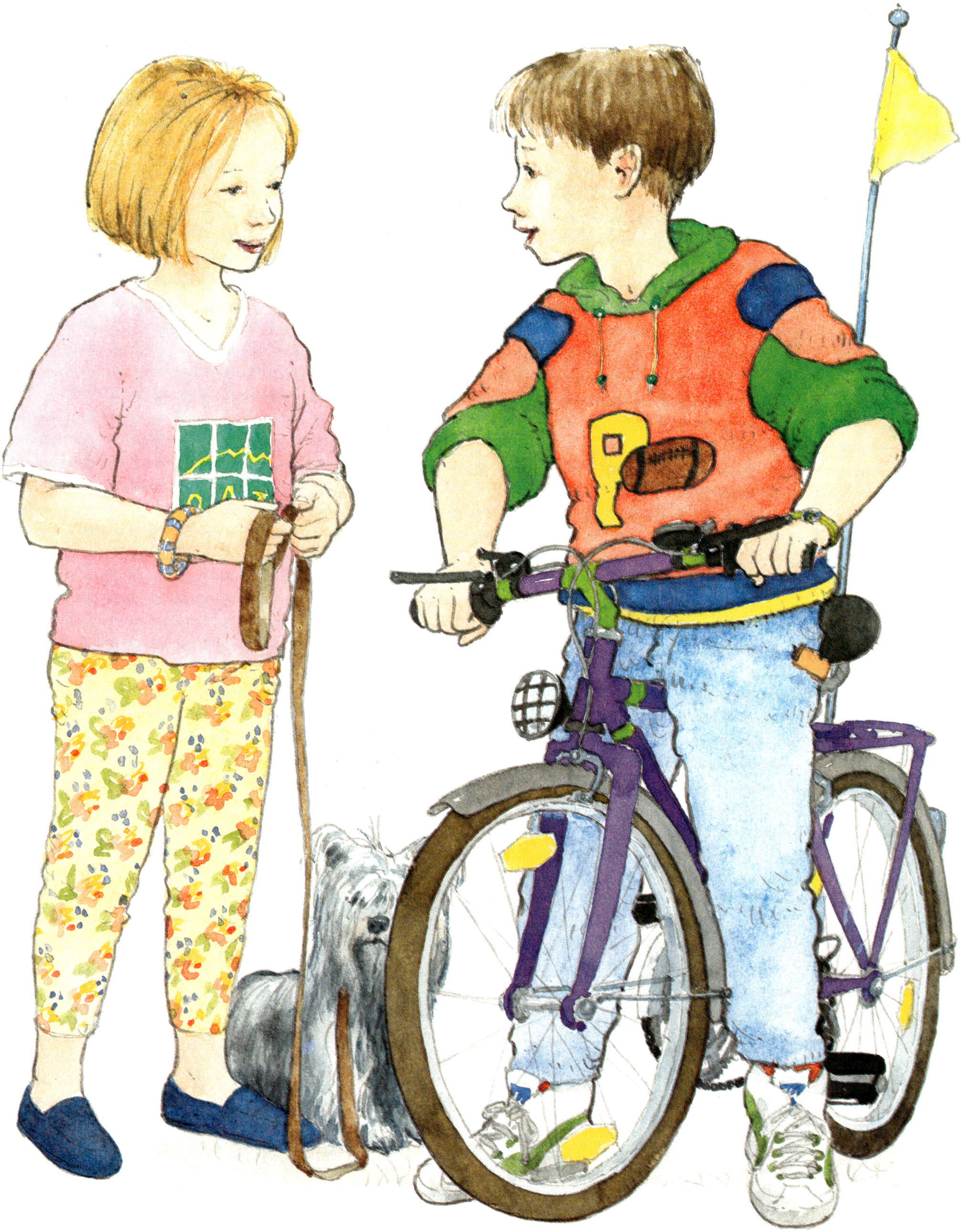

• How does the body control the levels of hormones it produces?

The hypothalmus, which lies at the base of the brain, controls the production of the hormones, testosterone, oestrogen and progesterone. Just as a thermostat ensures that the temperature in a room is kept constant, so the hypothalmus regulates the level of hormones in the bloodstream.
If the levels of testosterone in the blood are too high, for example, the hypothalmus slows down the production of the hormone until the levels have decreased.
In children of less than ten years old, the hypothalmus restricts the production of sexual hormones. During puberty, however, the production of such hormones is stimulated.
In boys, the production of testosterone is increased and in girls the production of oestrogen, in particular, is stepped up. The rise and fall in the amounts of these hormones in the body plays a very important part in reproduction.

• Where do sperm come from?

Inside each testicle are several compartments and in each compartment are many sperm tubules. The tubules are very narrow and, unrolled, they would measure about 500 metres long! The millions of cells lining the walls of these tiny tubes divide and develop into sperm. A sperm is made up of a head and a long tail which wiggles. The whiplash movement of the tail makes the sperm very mobile.
The sperms are collected from the tubules and stored in the epididymis. Eventually they move up the vas deferens to the seminal vesicle. This journey takes about two months.
The seminal vesicles and the prostate gland add fluids to the sperm as they pass through.
These fluids keep the sperm alive and allow them to swim. This mixture of sperm and fluid is known as semen. It is kept inside the body until the moment of ejaculation.

• What is ejaculation?

When a man has an erection, his penis swells and becomes firmer until it is quite hard. This is due to the mass of tissues inside the penis which have filled with blood.
When the penis has swollen to its full size, the foreskin is pulled back and the glans is exposed. If an erect penis is stimulated sufficiently, ejaculation takes place.
This is when semen shoots out of the penis in several jets.
An ejaculation is accompanied by an orgasm, which is a peaking of intense pleasure and sense of fulfilment.

• Can urine and sperm pass down the penis at the same time?

No, it is impossible for urination and ejaculation to happen at the same time. When a man is about to ejaculate, the bladder, in which urine is stored, is

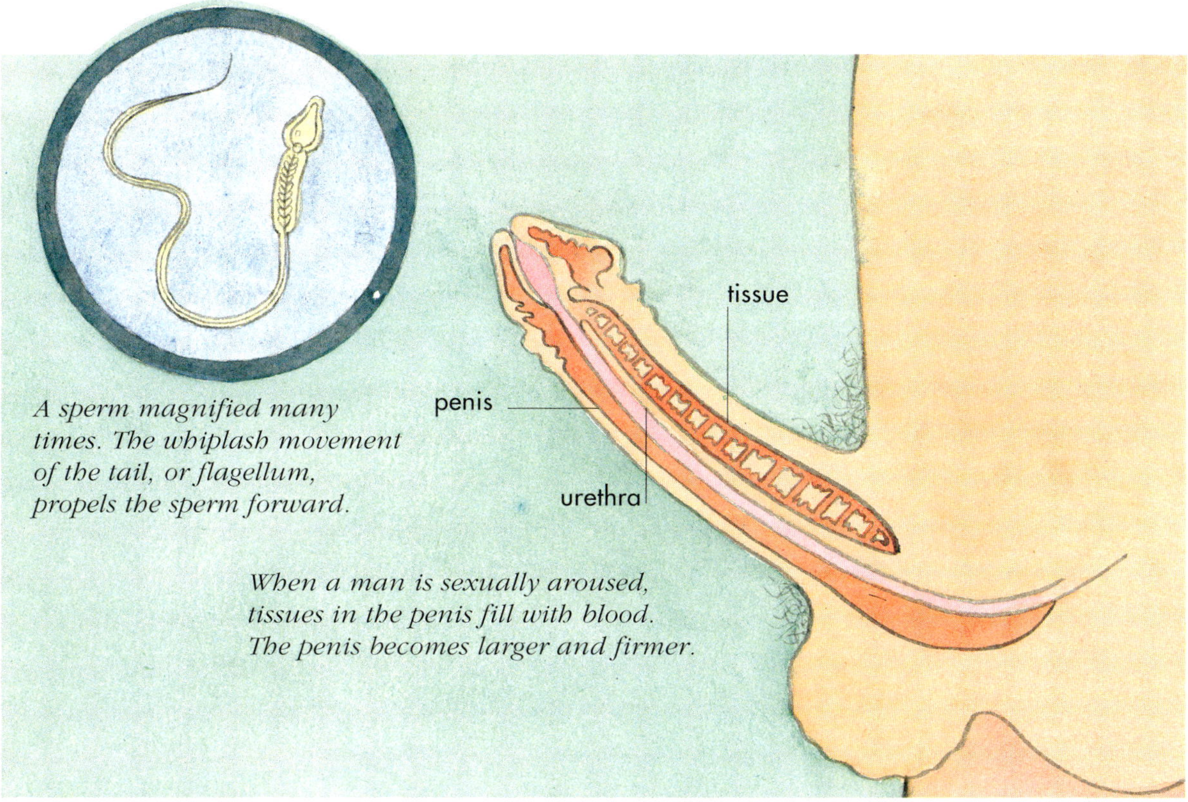

A sperm magnified many times. The whiplash movement of the tail, or flagellum, propels the sperm forward.

When a man is sexually aroused, tissues in the penis fill with blood. The penis becomes larger and firmer.

closed off by a flap which prevents urine from passing into the urethra and out of the penis.

• Is it true that penises need to be washed often?

The foreskin protects the glans from abrasion and drying out, but dirt and dead skin cells can be trapped beneath it. Apart from dirt and dead skin cells, a secretion called smegma also collects under the foreskin.

This must be removed by washing to avoid risk of infections, some of which can be quite painful in this area.

The foreskin is easily pulled back, however, to allow the glans to be washed with soap. If a man finds that his foreskin is too narrow or it sticks to the glans, he should see a doctor. A doctor may, in some cases, remove the foreskin. This is called circumcision.

Circumcision is a rite that is practised in certain religions, for example, Jews and Muslims are circumcised when they are still small boys.

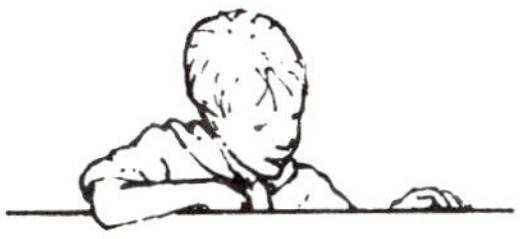

I am a Muslim. I was circumcised when I was a baby like all the other boys of my religion. But the Koran, the sacred book of Islam, does not mention circumcision. My Religious Education teacher says that we have probably adopted this practice from the Arabs, the Jews and the Egyptians.

Mohammed, 12 years old

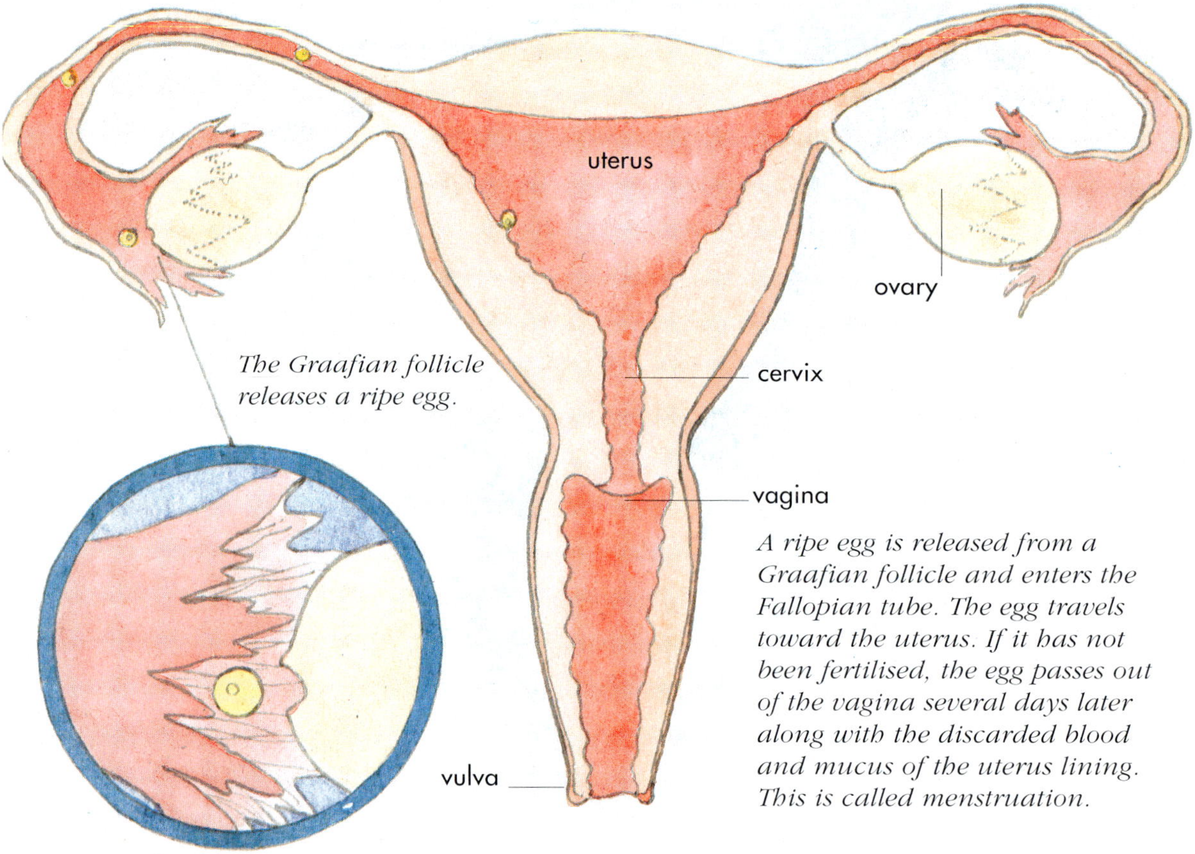

A ripe egg is released from a Graafian follicle and enters the Fallopian tube. The egg travels toward the uterus. If it has not been fertilised, the egg passes out of the vagina several days later along with the discarded blood and mucus of the uterus lining. This is called menstruation.

• Where do a woman's eggs come from?

Men start to produce sperm at the onset of puberty (at about 13-15 years old) and this continues throughout their lives. Women, however, do not wait until they are pubescent (10-12 years old) to start producing eggs. The eggs begin to form when a baby girl is still in her mother's womb. When a female baby is born, her ovaries already contain about 400,000 eggs and this number stays the same until menopause. At the onset of puberty, the ovaries are stimulated by changes in the levels of the hormones oestrogen and progesterone, into ovulation. This is when the ovaries release one egg between them every four weeks.

Eggs ripen at different times inside balls of cells called Graafian follicles. Several of the follicles, which lie on the surface of the ovaries, nourish an egg each until one of the eggs is ripe. At ovulation, the ripe egg bursts out of its follicle. It enters the Fallopian tube and is wafted towards the uterus.

Meanwhile, increased levels of progesterone have caused the lining of the uterus to thicken and become covered with mucus. If the egg is fertilised by a sperm on its way to the uterus, it will stick to this lining.

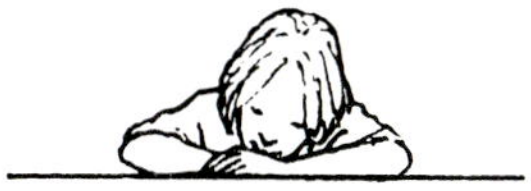

All the girls in my class have periods and they are very proud of the fact that they wear bras. I don't have either. I sometimes feel that I must be secretly younger than they are but the family doctor told me that I was just a late developer. He told me to be patient and that I would catch up one day soon. I wish my breasts would hurry up and grow so I can look more adult.

Helen 15 years old

What is puberty?

This is the period when a child's sexual organs develop. A boy's testicles begin to make sperm and a girl's ovaries cause eggs to ripen and be released. Other physical changes take place, such as the development of a girl's breasts and the growth of body hair under the arms and on the pubis.

• When does puberty begin?

Puberty begins at a slightly different time for each child. Girls generally enter puberty at the ages of 10 and 11. The first sign of puberty for them is the start of menstruation. In boys, puberty usually begins between the ages of 13 and 15. Other physical changes take place at different rates.
For example, a girl's breasts may develop early on so that by the age of 14 she will look physically mature, while the breasts of other girls may not be fully developed until the age of 17 or 18. Boys, too, develop at different rates and while one may have a mature penis by the age of 13, another may not reach this stage until he is 16 or 17.

• How often does menstruation take place?

Menstruation is when an unfertilised egg passes out of the uterus together with the blood that has been shed from the lining of the uterus. It takes several days to pass out through the vagina and this bleeding is commonly referred to as a period. A girl's first periods may be irregular, but after a while they occur once every four weeks.

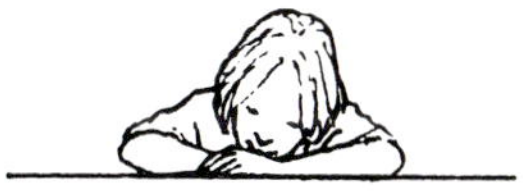

I started my periods about six months ago, but they are very irregular. Sometimes I go without one for two months. When I have my period I use sanitary towels and I always have lots of showers.

Julie, 13 years old

• What is the best sanitary protection during a period?

During a girl's period, she may either

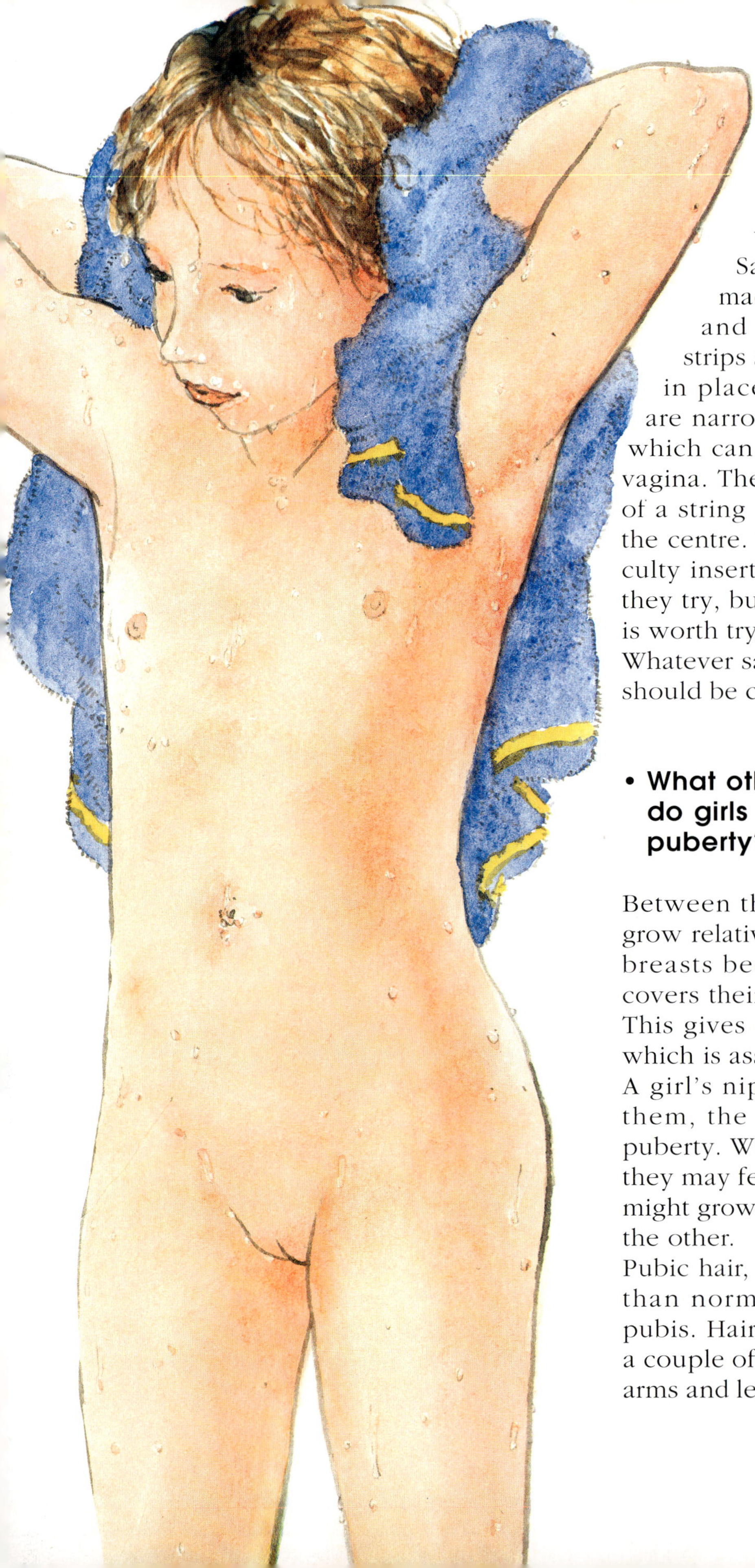

use a sanitary towel or a tampon. Sanitary towels are pads of cotton wool and other materials. Sanitary towels are specially made to fit closely to the body and most of them have sticky strips so that they remain securely in place in the panties. Tampons are narrow cylinders of cotton wool which can be inserted easily into the vagina. They are pulled out by means of a string which is firmly attached to the centre. Young girls may have difficulty inserting a tampon the first time they try, but this is quite natural and it is worth trying again at a later stage. Whatever sanitary protection is used, it should be changed regularly and often.

- **What other physical changes do girls experience during puberty?**

Between the ages of 10 and 14, girls grow relatively quickly in height. Their breasts become larger and extra fat covers their hips, thighs and buttocks. This gives them a more curved shape which is associated with femininity.

A girl's nipples and the area around them, the areola, also grow during puberty. While the breasts are growing they may feel lumpy or tender and one might grow slightly faster or larger than the other.

Pubic hair, which is curly, and coarser than normal hair, appears over the pubis. Hair under the armpits appears a couple of years later and hairs on the arms and legs become darker and longer. Girls will also start to find that their vagina is secreting a clear, slippery mucus between periods. This mucus is perfectly normal and there is not usually enough to worry about. If the secretion is pink or it gives off an unpleasant smell, it is advisable to see a doctor.

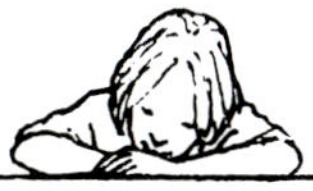

We often play netball at school. One day the ball hit my chest and my breasts hurt. My breasts are definitely more sensitive nowadays.

Mandy, 13 years old

• What are the effects of puberty on boys?

As in girls, a boy's rate of growth tends to increase rapidly during puberty and his testicles and penis fill out. At this time, the length of a boy's penis may differ from his friends' and this can cause jealousy. Boys with longer penises than others often feel they have the advantage over their friends, but in fact, the length of a penis is not important. It neither helps a boy to get a girlfriend nor improves his performance when making love.

The growth of the prostate gland and the epididymis is also stimulated at this time and the testicles start to produce sperm at a rate of several thousands of millions a year. A boy's first realisation

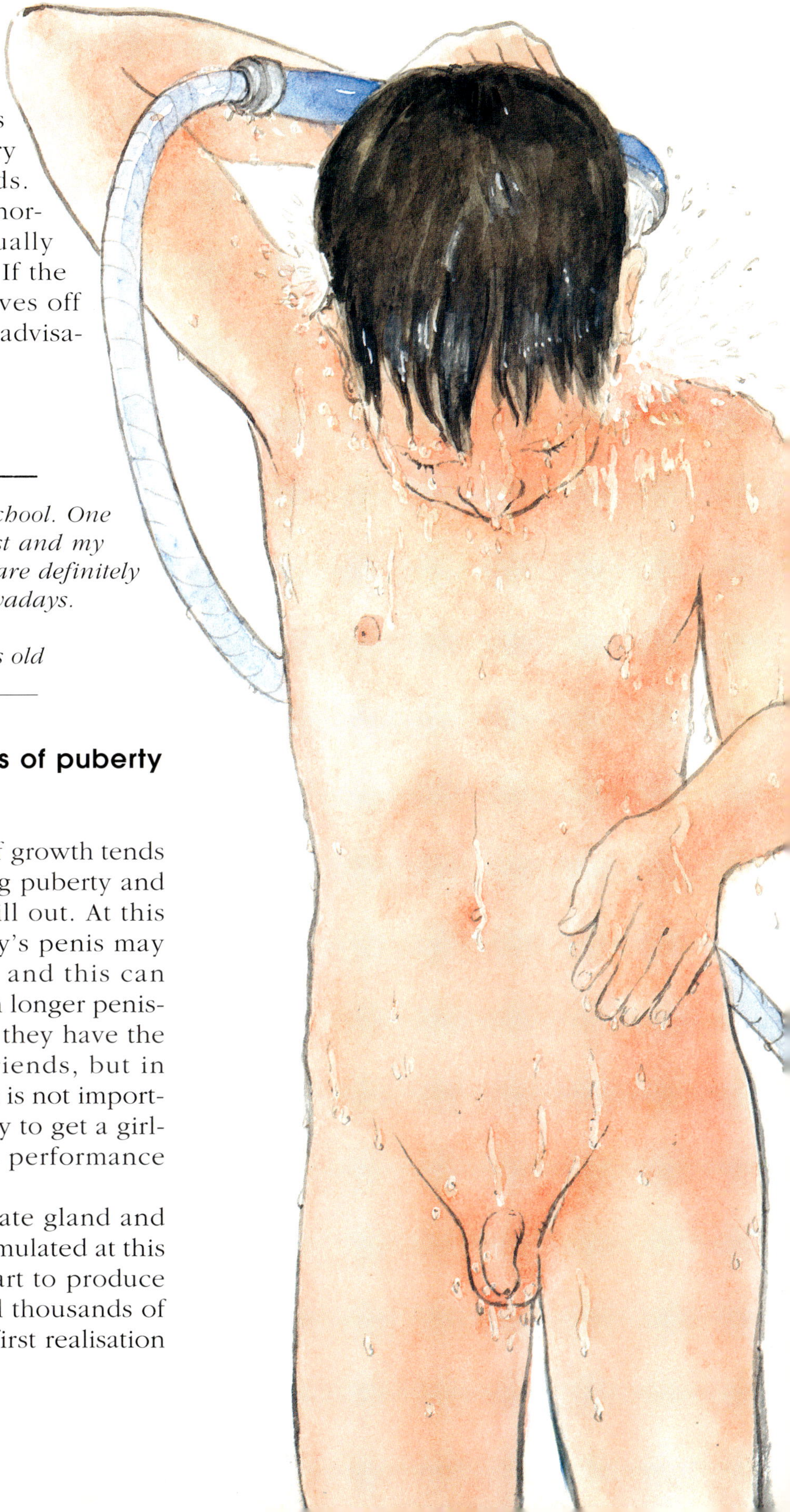

Body hair

Some children believe that women do not normally grow hair on their legs and arms! Many adolescent girls and women think that body hair looks ugly and should be removed. However, this hair is very natural and it is up to each individual as to whether and how it should be removed. Creams and razors are often used to remove hair (temporarily) from under armpits and legs. Hair on the arms, however, should not be shaved off, nor is it a good idea to remove pubic hair.

of this will probably be when he wakes up one morning to find he has ejaculated in his sleep. This is quite natural and most boys feel proud of this sign of manhood from their maturing bodies. Pubescent boys start to grow pubic hair around their penises and sometimes it grows from here in a line up to the navel. Hair thickens and darkens on the arms and legs and appears under the armpits.

Sweat glands become more active and body odour becomes noticeable.

During puberty, a boy's voice will deepen and after a couple of years, hair starts to grow on his upper lip, followed by the cheeks and chin. At first these hairs are quite fine, but they become thicker and coarser in time.

The relatively large amounts of testosterone in boys means that they develop larger muscles and denser bones than girls. Their muscles fill out during puberty and their body takes on a different shape to that of adolescent girls.

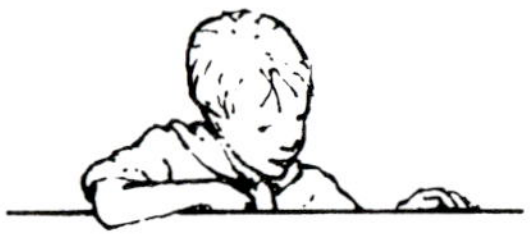

I hate music lessons because when I sing my voice cracks on some of the notes. I sing like a sick parrot now that my voice is breaking. Of course, my friends think it is very funny.

John, 14 years old

• Why do adolescents often have spots?

Many adolescents are afflicted with blackheads, red boils (acne) or pimples. The changing levels of hormones in boys and girls trigger sebum-producing glands and sweat glands. Sebum is an oily substance that covers the outer surface of the skin, keeping it supple and preventing it from drying out. Spots are caused by a blockage or the rupturing of these sebum-producing glands. All spots, especially acne, should be handled carefully. Although they are ugly to look at they disappear with time if left alone. Help and advice is always available from the leaflets that accompany the various skin care products at the chemist's.

The increased activity of sebum-producing glands also causes hair to become greasy more often. The same is true of the sweat glands in armpits. These are larger than ordinary sweat glands and

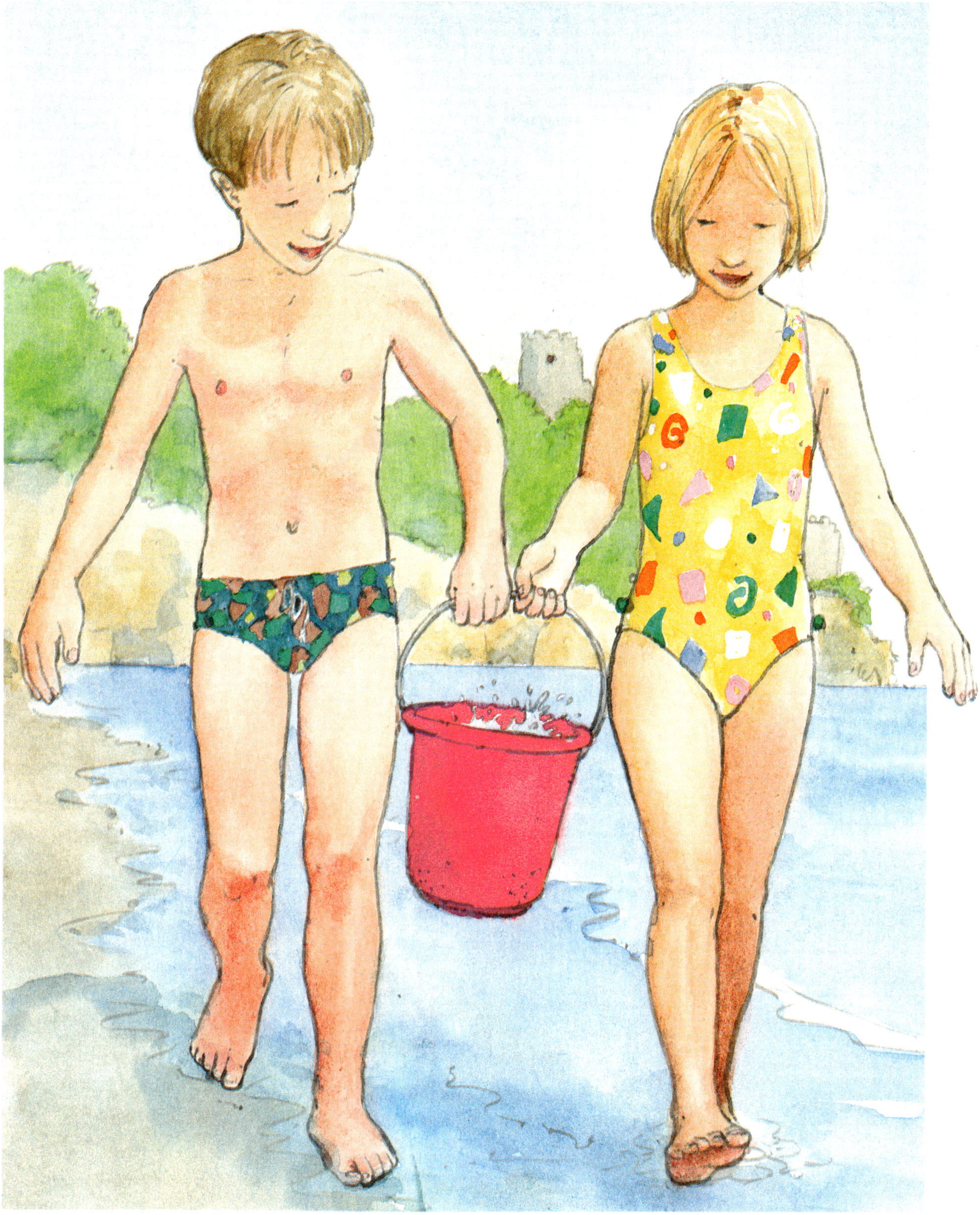

they produce more sweat. This sweat is acted on by bacteria in the air and broken down to cause the smell known as body odour. The simple solution to these problems is to wash often with soap.

• What other changes occur during puberty?

One of the most important effects of puberty is the self-awareness it brings to each individual. While changes are happening to the body, so changes are being made to an adolescent's way of thinking, behaving and feeling. Puberty is sometimes a traumatic time because so many changes are taking place at once. Teenagers begin to look inwards, developing their own ideas and opinions. At the same time they are given more responsibility and freedom to pursue their own desires. And this is the time when they are likely to fall in love.

Adolescents often feel the need to turn away from the family and spend time alone. They are determined to think and act for themselves. Some, indeed, go out of their way to establish their own identity and individuality. Unfortunately, this behaviour is often at the expense of the rest of the family who are hurt by what they feel is rejection. It is, ironically, at this precise time, when adolescents are trying to avoid communicating with their parents, that they most need advice and support to help them overcome the many challenges they are facing. Indeed most teenagers who want to break rules or ignore their parents' advice usually find they have to make their own when tempted by the freedom of the adult world which involves drugs, alcohol and sex. However, there are many advantages to puberty. Teenagers are given more freedom to do things as they want to or spend time with their friends.

Puberty can be a wonderful time: a time of fun, a time of discovery and excitement. It is also a time of change and confusion, of first love, happiness and pain.

• Is it wrong to masturbate?

It is natural for adolescents to want to touch their sexual organs. If they stroke them in a certain way they begin to feel a sort of excitement which increases until they experience a powerful sensation. This is called orgasm and in boys it is accompanied by ejaculation. Orgasm feels pleasurable, yet indescribable. Masturbation is the act of touching one's genitals until orgasm is reached. Most girls achieve this by touching or rubbing their clitoris. Boys rub or stroke their penises.

In the past, masturbation was considered dirty and wicked. Stories were told of people who masturbated and who were punished by becoming blind or growing hair on their palms.

Nowadays, masturbation is seen as part of growing up. It is just another way of finding out more about one's body.

A person who knows how his, or her, body is made and how it works will be better able to enjoy the act of making love.

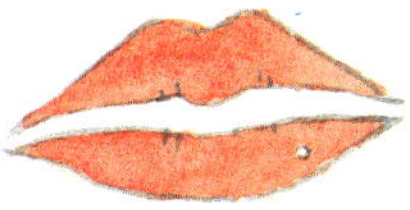
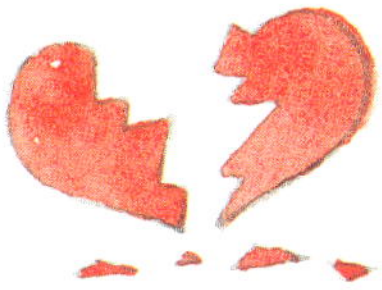
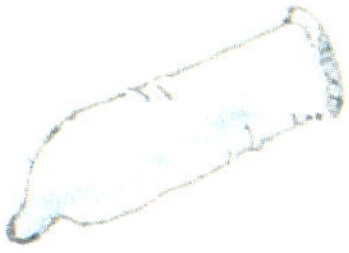
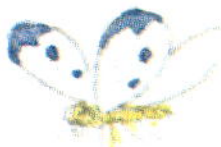
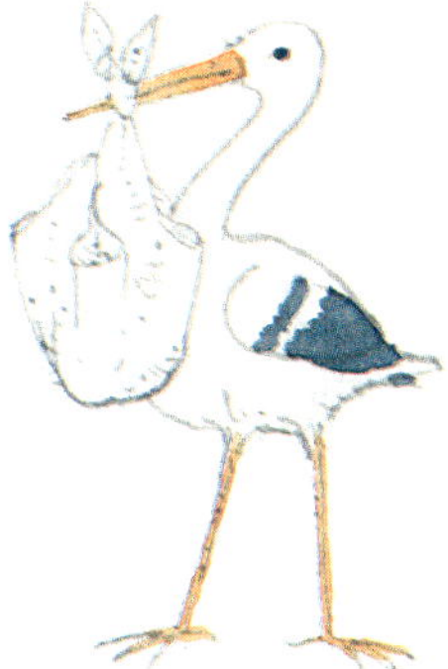

FERTILISATION

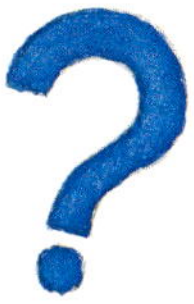

In the past, when either little was known about the internal workings of men and women, or when such issues were not talked about openly, reproduction was a mystery to most teenagers. They were told that babies were brought by storks or found under gooseberry bushes.
Many young women even got married without knowing the facts of life.
The following pages deal with fertilisation and the development of the embryo inside the womb, right up to the moment of birth.

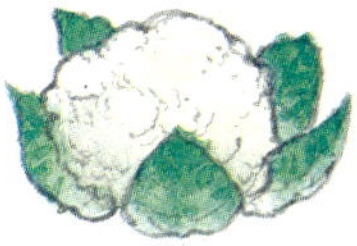
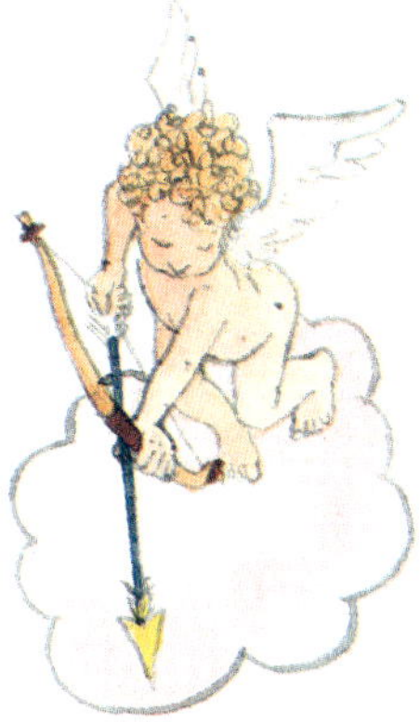
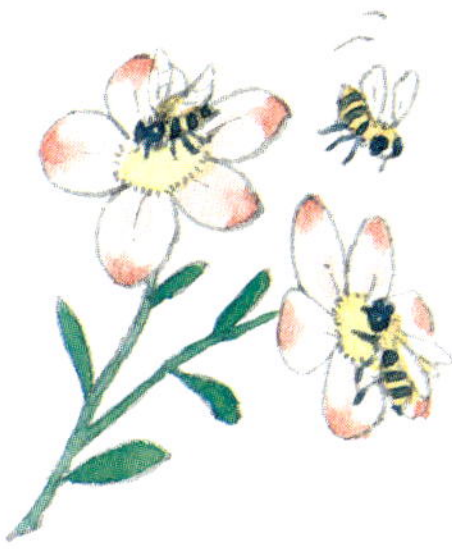
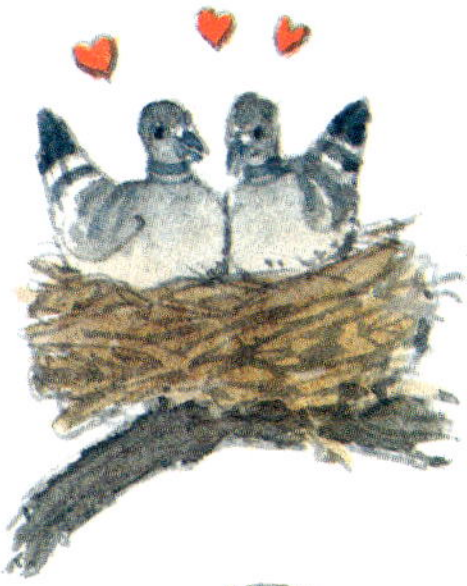
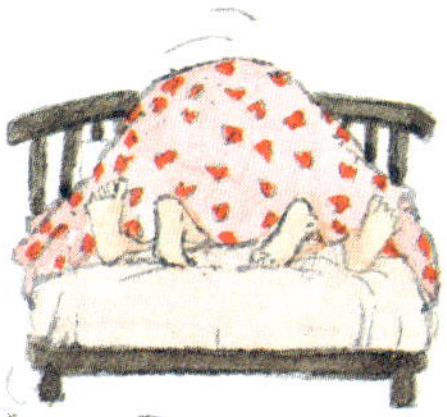
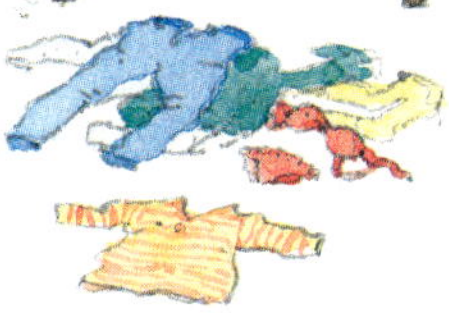
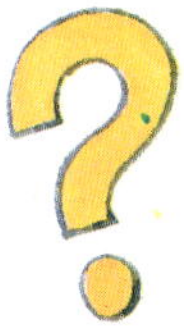

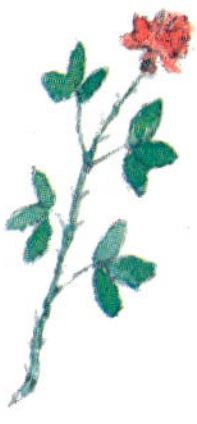
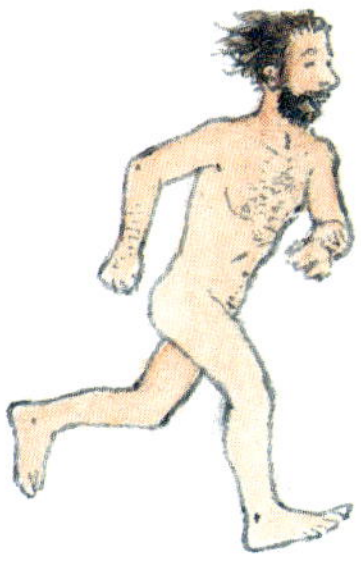
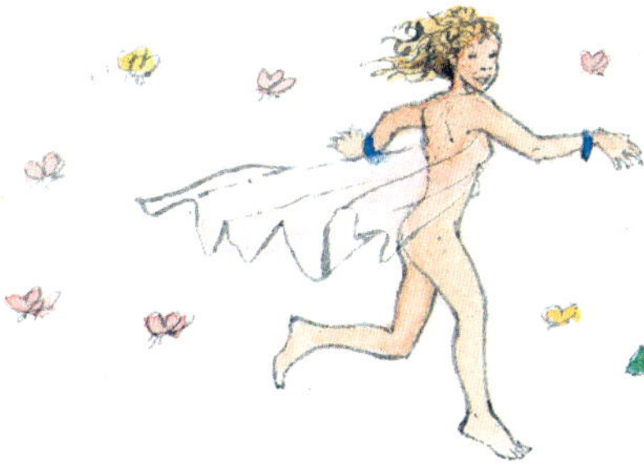
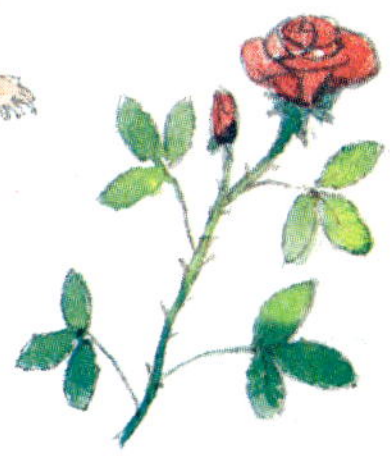

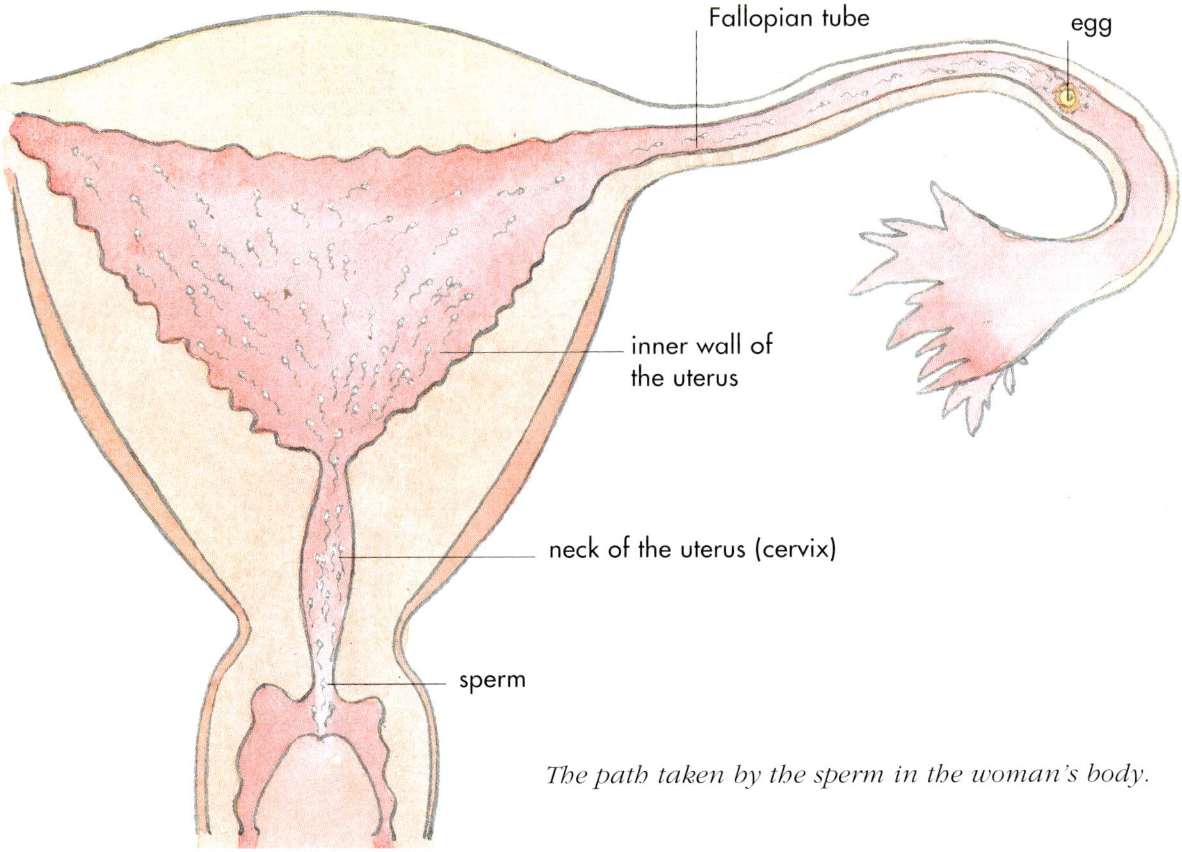

The path taken by the sperm in the woman's body.

• Where do the sperm and the egg meet?

When the egg leaves the ovary it moves down the Fallopian tube and towards the uterus. This journey takes several days.
In order for fertilisation to take place, the sperm and the egg have to meet and fuse together. About 400 million sperm are ejaculated into the vagina, but most of these do not pass through the cervix and others travel into the wrong Fallopian tube. The sperm that do survive the journey into the correct Fallopian tube live for between 48-72 hours. If an egg has already been released, the sperm cluster round it. Only one of these sperm is able to enter the egg and when it has done so the cell wall hardens, thus preventing any others from following. The two cells fuse together to become one and the egg is fertilised. The cell, which is now called an embryo, starts to divide as it moves towards the uterus with its thick wall lining of blood and mucus.

• What happens to the fertilised egg in the uterus?

When the ball of rapidly dividing cells reaches the uterus it attaches itself to the wall, usually in the top third.
Special cells on its surface burrow into

1

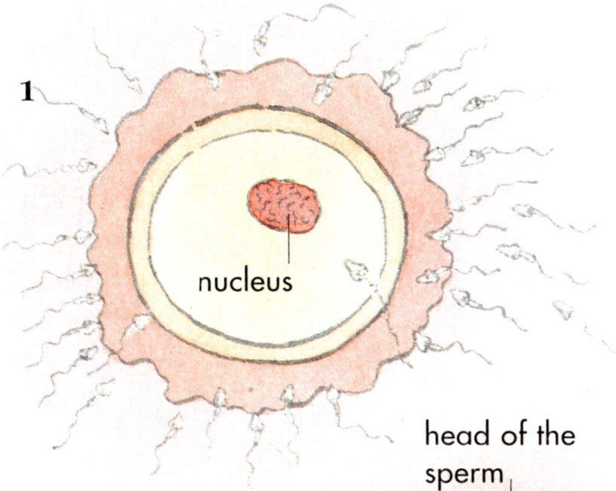

A week's journey

Four days after fertilisation, the egg arrives in the uterus where it attaches itself to the wall. After about three days, the embryo sinks into the lining of the uterus. Once embedded in the lining it takes nine months for the baby to grow.

2

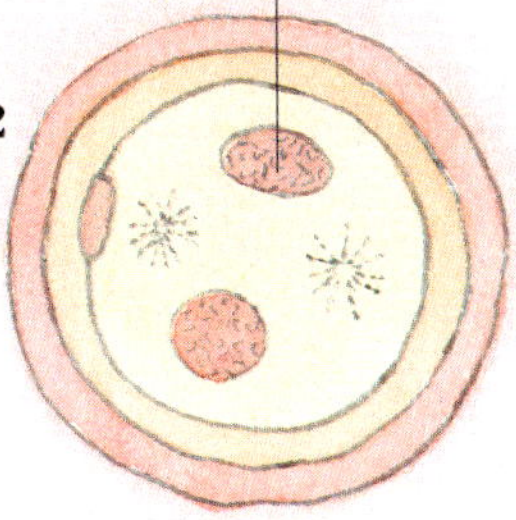

the lining. This is comparable to a seed which falls on fertile soil and grows roots which both support it and take in water and minerals. The embryo taps into blood vessels in the uterus wall and begins to form its own minute blood vessels. Eventually the placenta is formed here.

3

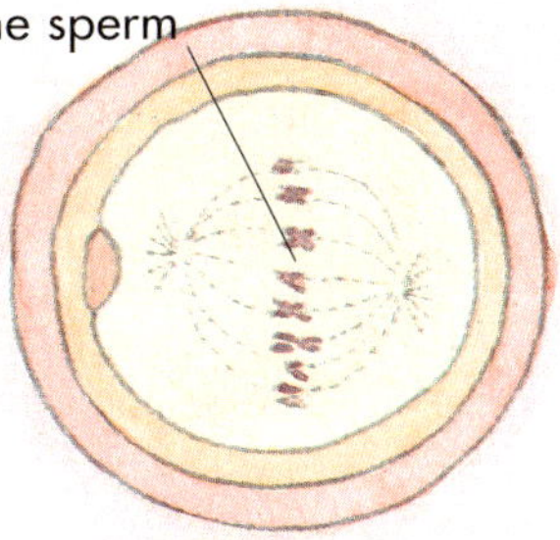

1. *The egg is a cell which contains a nucleus with 23 chromosomes. A single sperm penetrates the cell wall and loses its tail as it does so.*
2. *The head of sperm, which also contains 23 chromosomes, enlarges.*
3. *The chromosomes of both egg and sperm meet and pair off. The fertilised egg now contains 46 chromosomes.*
4. *Further sperm are prevented from entering the egg by the layers of jelly which surround it and which become thicker and harder.*
5. *The egg starts to divide, first into two. Each cell has 46 chromosomes. The egg is now called an embryo.*

• Will the baby be a boy or a girl?

The sperm and the egg each contain 23 chromosomes, each of which carries messages about what sort of person the embryo will become. Chromosomes determine a person's height, gender, hair colouring, eye colouring and so on. As soon as a sperm and an egg have joined, the gender of the baby is decided. An egg contains a sex chromosome which is always an X.
A sperm, on the other hand, may have

4

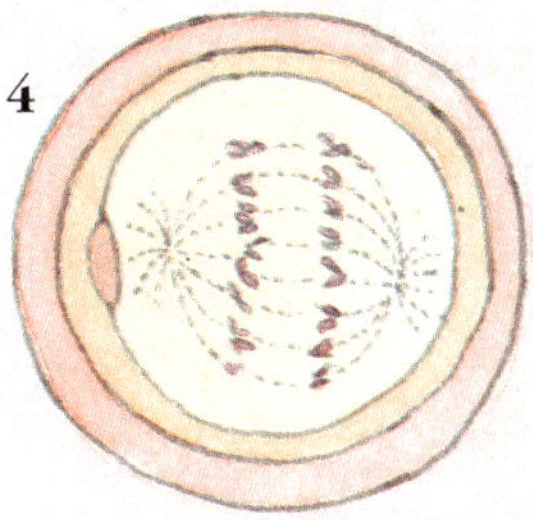

5

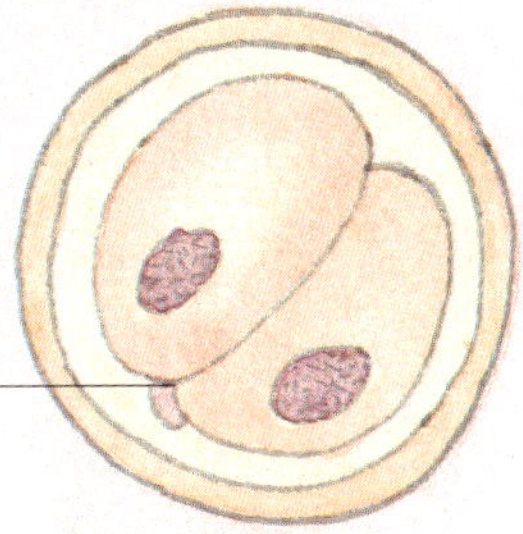

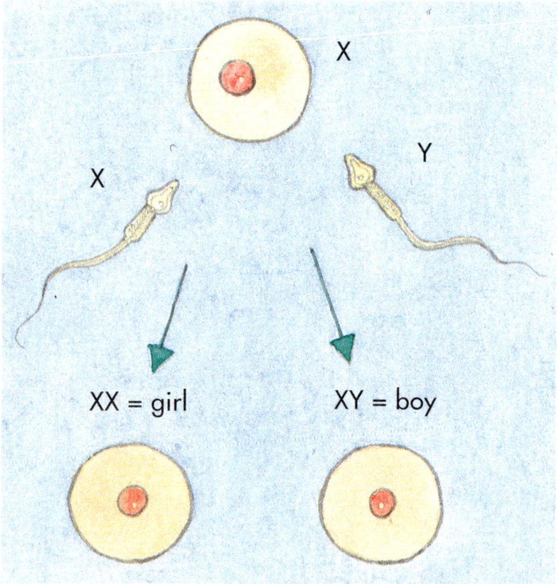

One of the man's 23 chromosomes determines the gender of the baby

either an X or a Y chromosome. X chromosomes make females and Y chromosomes make males. If the embryo has two X chromosomes, it will become a girl, but if it has an X and a Y chromosome, it will develop into a boy. It is, therefore, the sperm which determines the sex of the baby.
The embryo has 46 chromosomes. If there are any fewer or any more, the child may be deformed in some way.

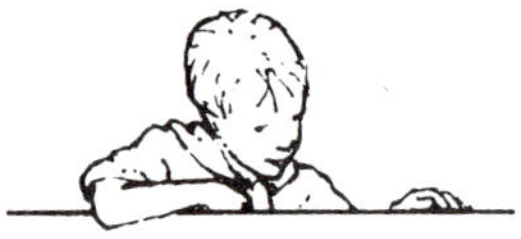

Our neighbour gave birth to her fourth child when she was 45 years old. The baby had Down's Syndrome. Mummy says that the chances of having a baby with Down's Syndrome increase with age for women who are over 30 years old.

Matthew, 12 years old

• Why is each being unique?

Chromosomes determine everything about us, even, to some extent, our personalities. The chromosomes from the woman merge with the chromosomes of the man to make up a totally new human being.
For example, if the mother's chromosome determining eye colour is brown while that of the father is blue, only one of these can be chosen. Because the chromosome for brown eyes is always dominant over blue, the child will have brown eyes. The child will, therefore, look like one of his parents or his grandparents. The child will inherit some of his parents' features and some of their parents', thus creating a totally new combination of features.

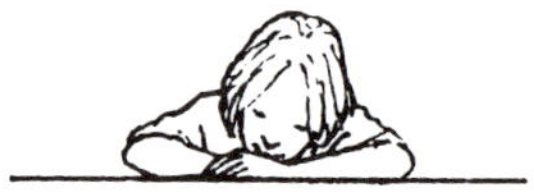

I never knew my grandmother. She died when I was still a baby. My mother tells me that she was an extremely obstinate woman. Both my parents say that I have inherited this characteristic. I'm afraid they're right!

Sophie, 13 years old

• How does the growth of an embryo start?

As soon as the fertilised cell of 46 chromosomes is formed, it begins to divide. The cells divide and divide again, doubling the number of new cells each time. The chromosomes give instruc-

We look and think the same!

Identical twins are often so alike that it is difficult to tell them apart.
They may even be able to guess what each other is thinking or about to say. They are often ill at the same time.

tions to the cells so that they become different organs, tissues and other parts of the body.

• What are identical twins?

Most women give birth to just one baby, but sometimes they have two babies at once. This happens when a fertilised egg splits in two. The information carried by the chromosomes is duplicated and the two embryos develop into identical twins.

The embryos both have exactly the same chromosomes which means

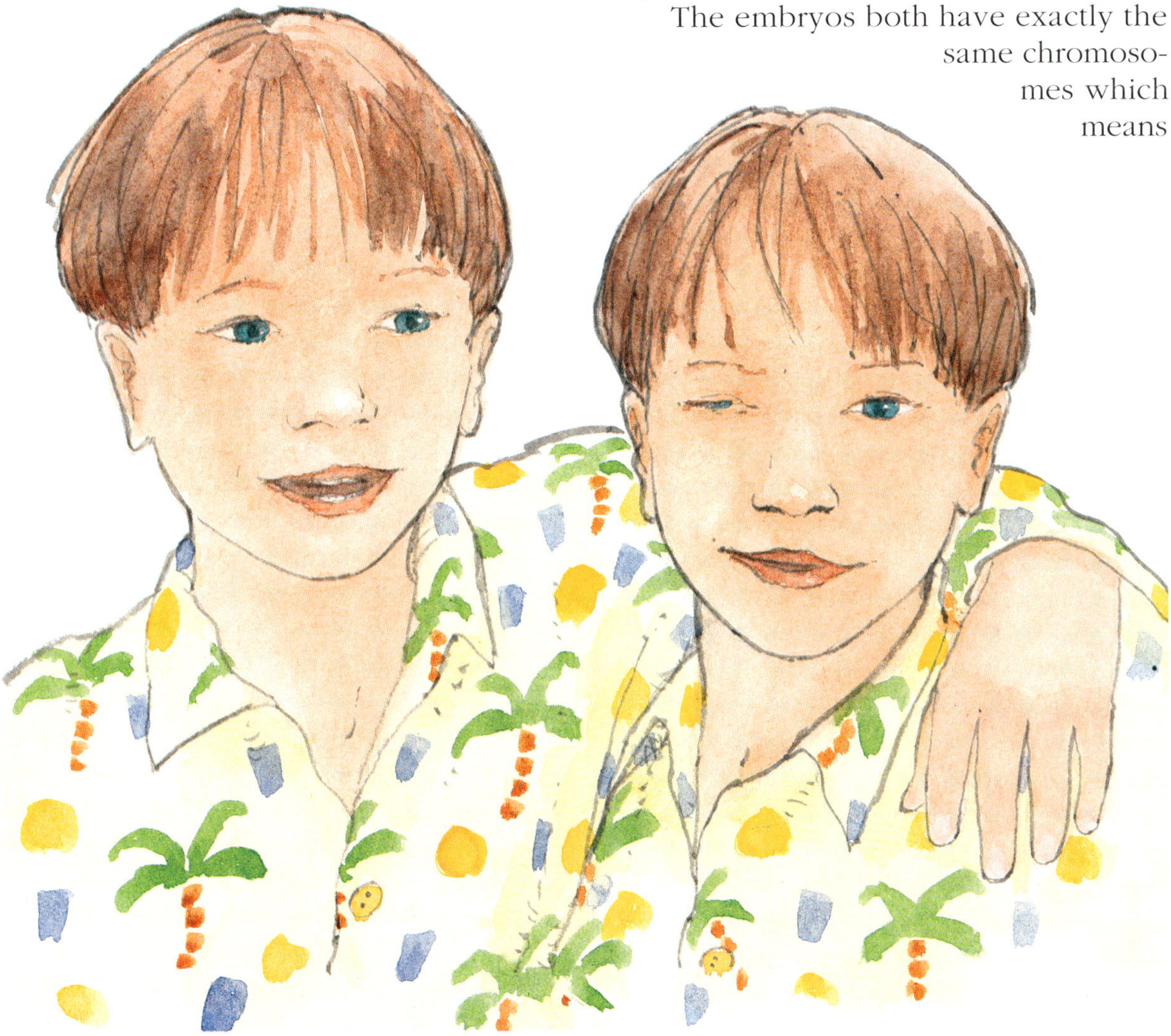

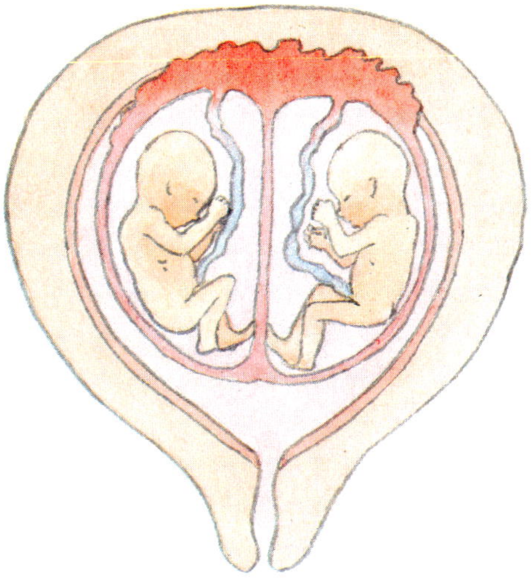

identical twins

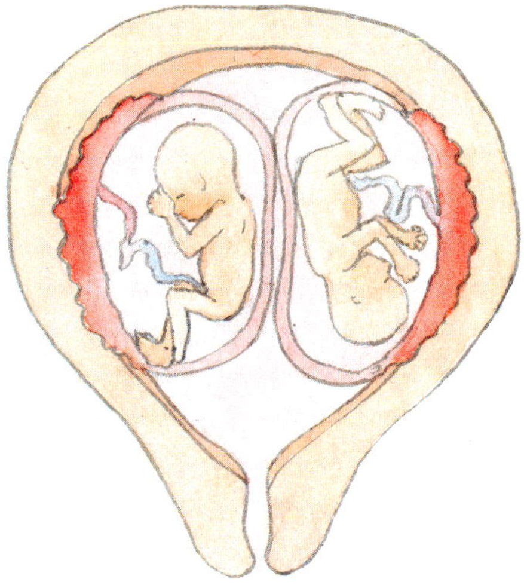

fraternal twins

that they will be of the same gender and they will look and behave like each other.
The twins even share the same placenta in the uterus.

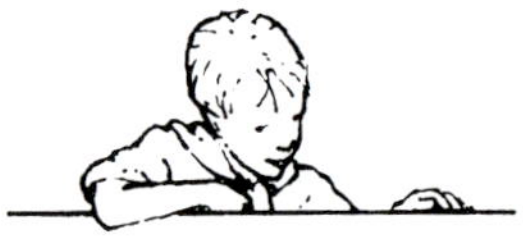

There are a pair of identical twins in my class. Sarah and Julie look so like each other that you can't tell them apart. They are also alike in other ways. For example, they are both brilliant at maths and terrible at games.

Peter, 12 years old

• What are fraternal twins?

If an ovary releases two eggs at the same time, it is possible that both of them will be fertilised. Each egg is fertilised by a different sperm and in this case the children are no more alike than if they were ordinary brothers and sisters.
Unlike identical twins, who share the same placenta, fraternal twins each have a separate supply of blood and food from the mother.

• What is the likelihood of multiple births?

A multiple birth is when a woman gives birth to triplets, quadruplets and so on. Multiple births are very rare and they are usually a result of taking fertility drugs rather than a hereditary characteristic. Fertility drugs are taken when a woman is having problems becoming pregnant. The drug causes several eggs to ripen in the Graafian follicles and be released at once.
If the ripe eggs are fertilised there will be several embryos in the uterus at the same time.
When they are born the babies are often frail and very small.

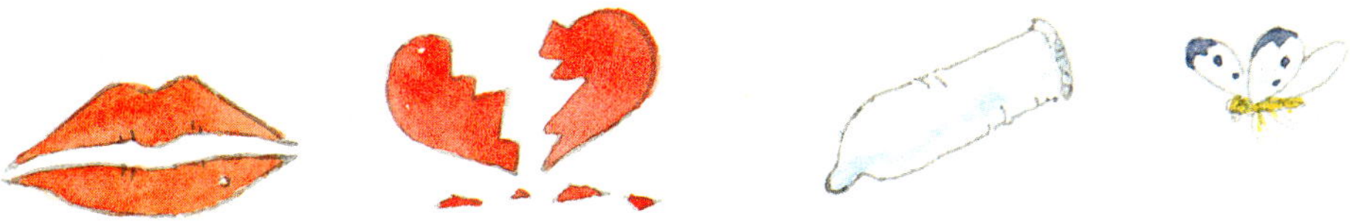

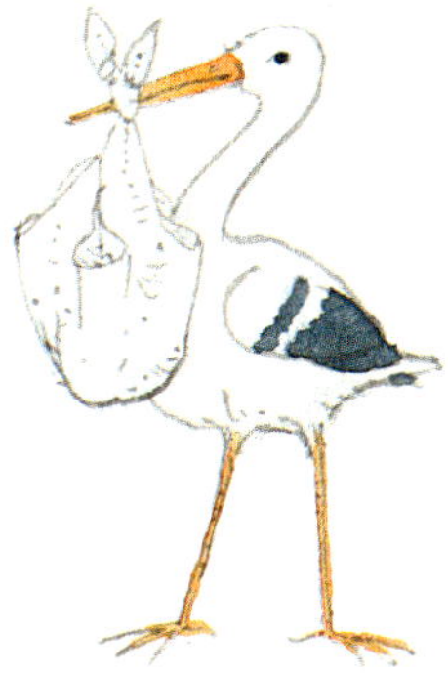

MAKING LOVE

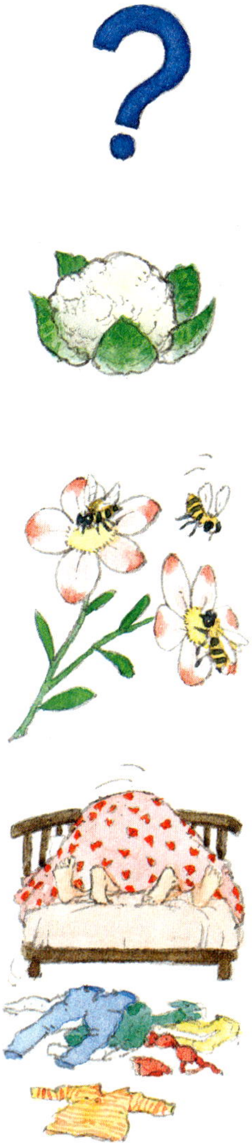

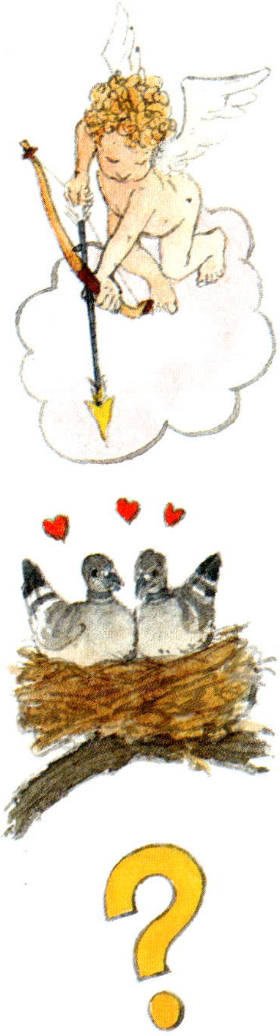

When a person falls in love, it is because they are attracted to the looks and personality of another person.

If two people are attracted to each other they will want to spend all their free time together getting to know each other. They will become good friends and, by trusting, supporting and protecting one another, they will become very close. At some point in the relationship they will cuddle, kiss and explore each other's bodies.

Caressing and fondling will often lead on to making love (sexual intercourse).

All couples make love in the way that best suits them. A man may lie on top of the woman or she may position herself on top of him. There are many positions to experiment with.

Not all couples who make love are necessarily in love. It may be just a natural response to a physical attraction which, in time, wears off.

However, it is when a couple develop a relationship that goes further than mere physical attraction that they feel a greater satisfaction in making love with someone they know well and care for.

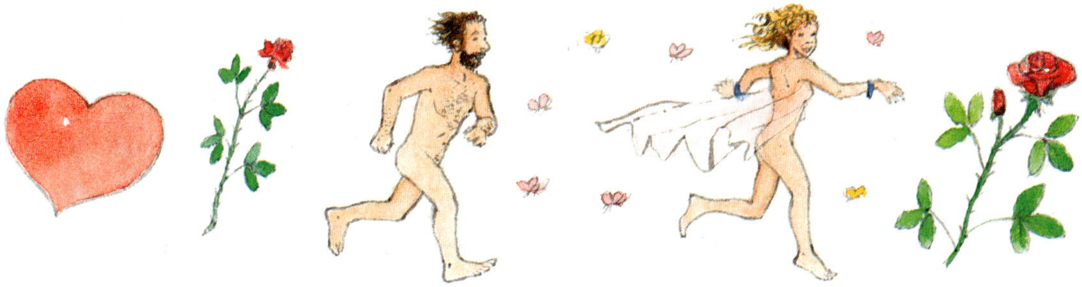

• How do the sperm and egg meet?

When two people in love kiss and caress each other they become aroused. For those who have had little or no experience of sexual intercourse this is a powerful sensation.

Arousal occurs through being touched on the external sexual organs and erogenous zones. These are areas which give particular pleasure if they are stroked or touched. Apart from being touched on the penis and the scrotum, for example, men may like to have their nipples kissed or earlobes nibbled. Women are aroused by fondling of the breasts, nipples and clitoris.

There are many erogenous zones to be discovered for each individual.

When a man or woman is aroused, certain things start to happen to their bodies. A man's penis enlarges and becomes hard. It sticks up against his lower belly and the glans becomes moist and slippery. The woman's nipples harden and her vagina becomes longer. It secretes a mucus that lubricates it.

When a couple are sexually aroused, they will probably want to make love. When they do so, the man will put his erect penis into the woman's vagina and move it back and forth rhythmically. This stimulation of the penis is an enjoyable sensation for the man.

The woman will also feel pleasure from the man's movements, especially if her clitoris is being touched. When the stimulation has reached a peak, the man's penis will ejaculate semen. At the same time as ejaculation the man will feel intense pleasure and if the woman has climaxed at the same time she will experience a similar sensation. This is an orgasm.

An orgasm causes the woman's cervix to open slightly and the uterus to contract in order to draw the sperm into it. The sperm travel into the uterus on their way to meeting an egg (if one has been released).

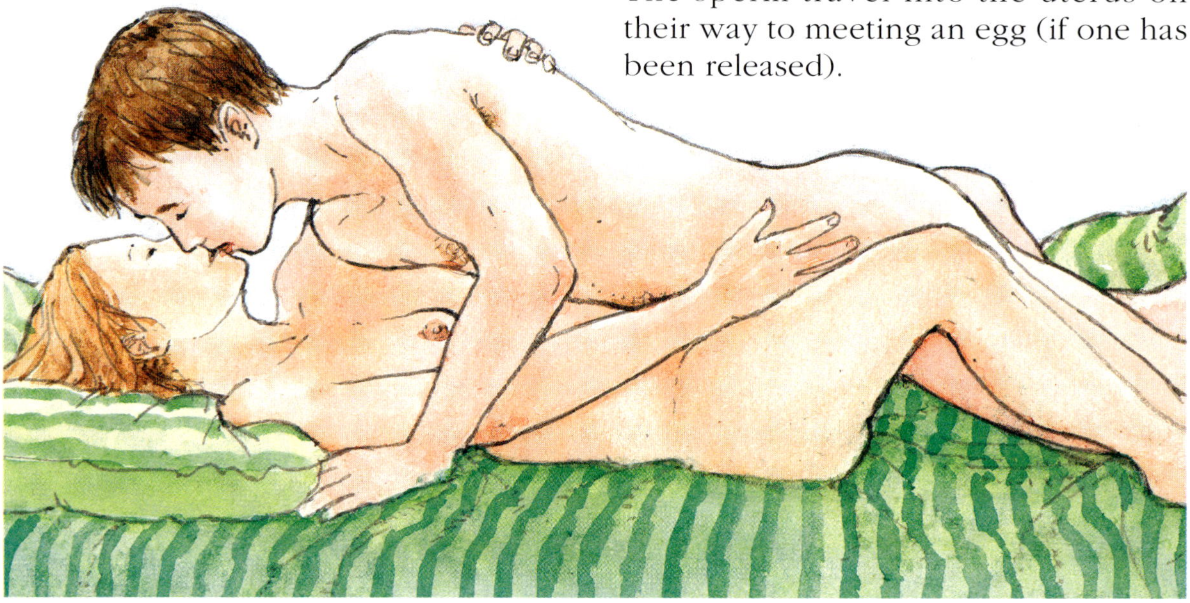

• **How is it possible to avoid getting pregnant after making love?**

The attraction of man and woman to one another is completely natural. It is nature's way of survival, of continuing the species. However, women nowadays do not have to run the risk of becoming pregnant each time they make love and mothers rarely have more than four children because they use contraception. There are many types of contraception, some natural and some medical.

A natural, but relatively risky form of contraception is the rhythm method. There are only a few days each month during which ovulation occurs. An egg is released at this time and a woman can become pregnant. If her periods are regular she can estimate that 14 days after the start of her last period is the time when it is unsafe because the egg has been released.

This method is slightly less risky if she takes her temperature every day. At the time of ovulation her body temperature will rise by a few degrees and if she makes a careful record of her temperature in the form of a chart she can see when to avoid making love.

Another type of rhythm method is to check the state of the cervical mucus. This method must be clearly explained by a doctor, however, before it is attempted.

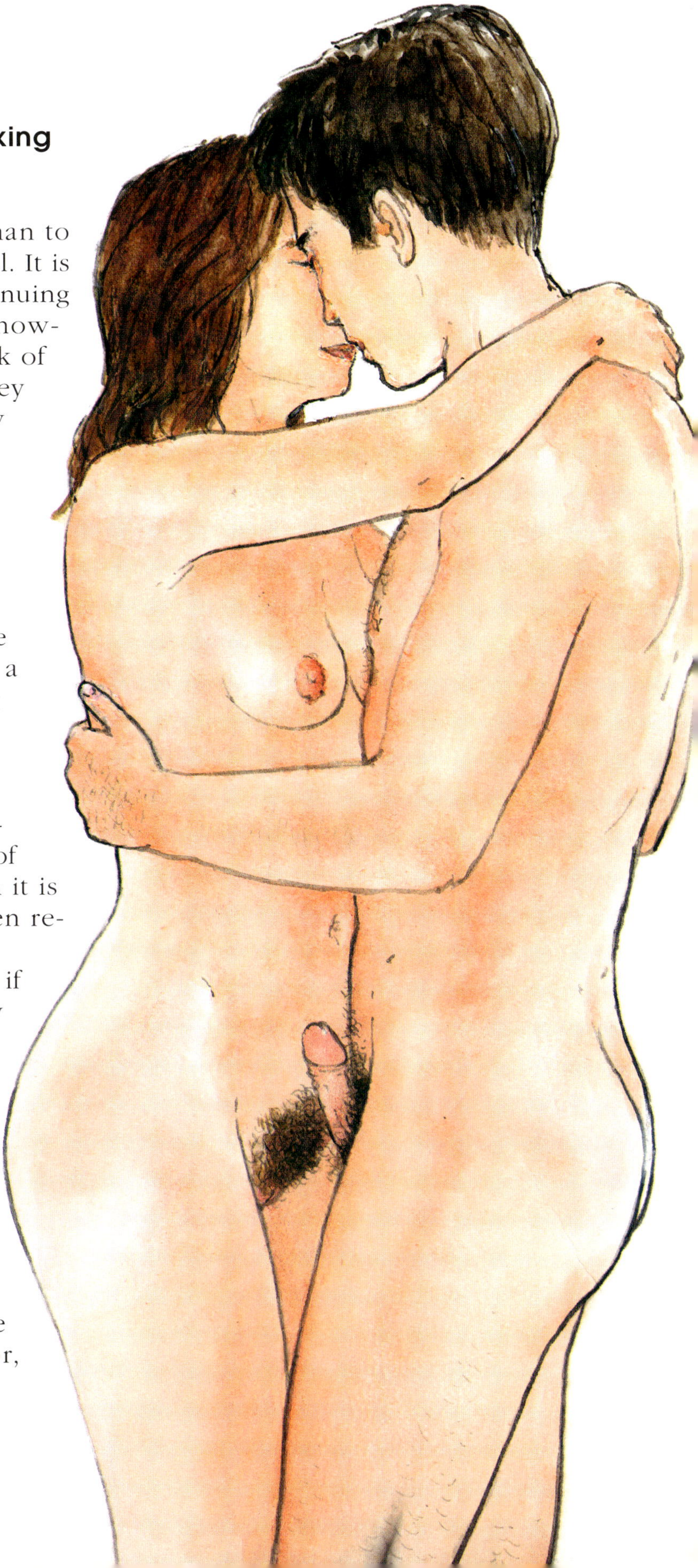

How does a woman know if she is pregnant?

- Her periods stop.
- Her breasts become tender.
- She may feel sick without really being ill.
- Her eating habits change.
- She has to urinate more often.
- She feels tired.
- Some women find they have a strange taste in their mouth.
- Others cannot drink tea or coffee.

A pregnancy test involves putting a few drops of blood or urine into a special liquid. It is a more reliable way of finding out than waiting to see if a missed period is due to pregnancy.
Pregnancy test kits can be bought in chemist's shops and used at home.

Clearly these methods are not risk free. Ovulation may be early or late for many reasons and body temperatures may rise and fall due to illness.
An even more unreliable method of natural contraception is the withdrawal method.
This is when the man withdraws his penis from the woman's vagina just before ejaculation.
This method is very unsatisfactory. The woman will probably feel frustrated because she has not had an orgasm and there is the very real worry that some sperm have been released from the penis before ejaculation.
This is why most couples use other types of contraception which have to be taken or used before intercourse, but which are much safer.
Many young women take the Pill, while others use a coil or cap.
Men protect women from becoming pregnant by wearing condoms.

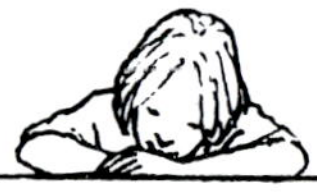

One of the girls in my class is going out with a boy who is 17 years old. She has told me that they make love and he uses a condom. I don't feel I am ready to go that far with a boy yet. It would make me feel uncomfortable. Anyway, there is plenty of time for that sort of thing later.

Anna, 15 years old

• What happens when a woman takes the Pill?

The Pill controls the amounts of the sexual hormones progesterone and oestrogen in the woman's body.
Reduced hormone levels prevent the ovaries from producing eggs. If there is no egg, there cannot be a pregnancy.
The mini-Pill contains only one hormone which thickens the cervical mucus, thus preventing sperm from getting through.
It also makes it more difficult for the uterus to accept a fertilised egg. This pill only works if it is taken at almost exactly the same time each day.

• Which contraceptive is the safest?

The Pill is usually considered the safest contraceptive if it is taken correctly and the woman has not been sick after taking it.

Condoms are particularly useful for couples who have formed a relationship in a short time and where the woman has either not had time to go on the Pill or it has not yet taken effect.

Condoms are thin rubber tubes which are rolled down over the man's penis when it is erect. A spermicidal cream may be also be placed in the woman's vagina. When the man ejaculates, the semen is caught in the nipple-shaped end of the condom. Provided the condom is removed before the penis shrinks back to its normal size, none of the sperm should have entered the woman's vagina.

The combination of condom and spermicidal cream is probably as reliable as the Pill and they are a particularly good method of contraception because they prevent one partner infecting the other with a venereal disease or AIDS.

A condom, if used correctly, protects against AIDS

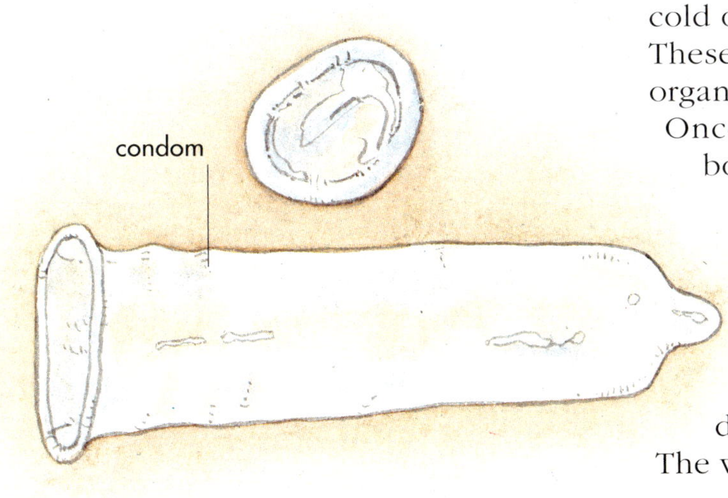

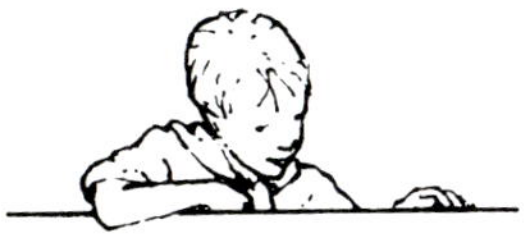

One of my friends brought a condom to school. We went to the toilets and filled it up with water. You should have seen the amount of water it took to fill it! They must be very strong - it stretched until it was big enough to fit around a man's wrist.

William, 15 years old

• What is AIDS?

AIDS stands for Acquired Immune Deficiency Syndrome. It is a disease that causes the person it has infected to lose the ability to fight infection.

Eventually the sufferer becomes very ill and dies.

At school each day there are probably one or two people with sore throats, a cold or the beginnings of flu.

These infections are caused by microorganisms, such as bacteria or viruses. Once the invaders have entered the body they attack the system. However, they are prevented from causing too much harm by white platelets, a type of blood cell. If the white platelets are not successful, another type of cell, called a T cell, helps to destroy the invader.

The white cells and the T cells are part

of the immune system.
A person who has AIDS cannot fight the body's invaders effectively. HIV (Human Immunodeficiency Virus) the virus that causes AIDS attacks the immune system and damages the T cells. This leaves an AIDS sufferer open to all infections and diseases.
Infections that would otherwise be fought off within a couple of days develop into illnesses that last longer and cause more harm than usual. Even a common cold can become pneumonia and lead to death.
People most at risk from AIDS are homosexual men.
However, some of these men are bisexual, which means they have sexual intercourse with both men and women. Bisexual men are, therefore, able to infect heterosexual women who, in turn, infect other men, and so the disease spreads.

Scare stories which are not true

There are all sorts of scare stories about AIDS which cause more harm than good. For example, no, you will not get AIDS if you touch someone who is infected with the HIV virus; nor if you share their plate or glass.
Some people worry that they will catch AIDS from a mosquito bite. This is also untrue. The HIV virus is transmitted via blood, semen and vaginal fluids.

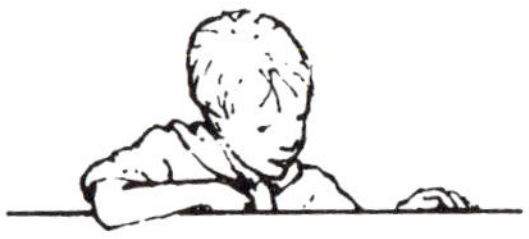

I have slept with several girls and I always use a condom. I am enjoying life too much to risk getting AIDS or a sexually transmitted disease. Some of my mates don't take any precautions. I mean, they don't use a condom because they say the girl is on the Pill. They know about AIDS as well as I do, but they think it is less macho. I can't understand them, it's their life they're playing with.

Mick, 19 years old

• How can AIDS be avoided?

The AIDS virus is caught through contact with infected blood, semen and vaginal fluids.
It is possible, therefore, to catch it by making love with someone who has been infected. The only way to avoid this is by using a condom when making love. Semen is contained inside the condom and prevented from coming into contact with the partner's body fluids or blood.
The AIDS virus can live in the body for several years without the victim developing full-blown AIDS. Furthermore, AIDS has spread alarmingly over the last decade and many of those who have been infected will not realise it. So it is wise to continue using a condom for a few years into a relationship or until both partners have taken an AIDS test. Women whose partners refuse to wear a condom are advised to wear a female condom (see p. 35).

• Can AIDS be caught in other ways?

Unfortunately, many people have caught AIDS after a blood transfusion with infected blood. Before much was known about AIDS, donated blood was not screened and some of it was infected. Nowadays, however, all donated blood in this country is screened for the AIDS virus. AIDS can also be caught from an unsterilised hypodermic needle. Drug addicts often use such needles when injecting drugs into their bodies. Sadly, pregnant addicts who have become infected with the virus have given birth to babies which already have the virus in their system.

• What are the other contraceptives?

Some women, usually those who have had babies, use a coil or IUD (Intra-uterine-contraceptive Device). This is a small piece of plastic that is put inside the uterus by a doctor. The coil is very effective but it can cause heavy periods and occasional stomach cramps.

The cap, or diaphragm, is popular with some women. It is a circle of rubber with a springy rim and it has to be fitted by a doctor who measures the correct size.

The cap is placed across the top of the vagina or over the cervix. The woman inserts it before love-making, together with a spermicidal cream.

A similar device to the cap is the female condom. This looks like a cross between a condom and a cap. It is placed in the vagina before making love. The female condom has only recently been

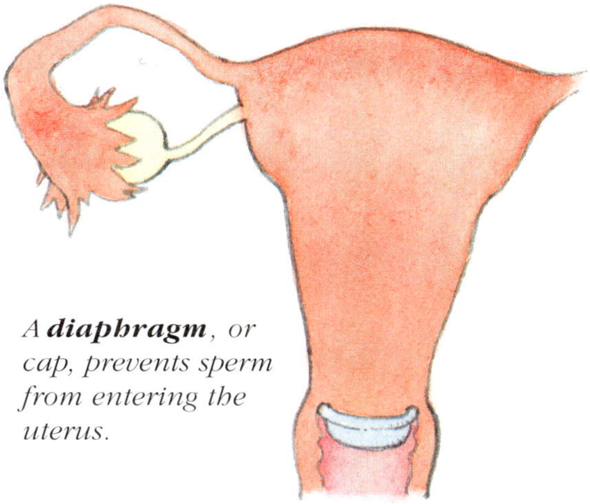

*A **diaphragm**, or cap, prevents sperm from entering the uterus.*

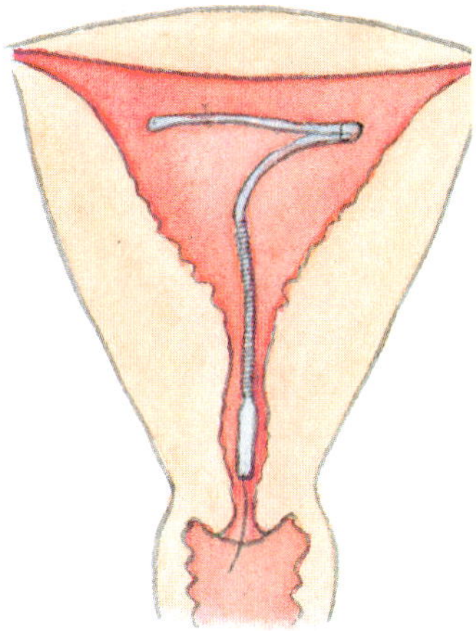

*The **coil**, or IUD, deters eggs from attaching themselves to the uterus.*

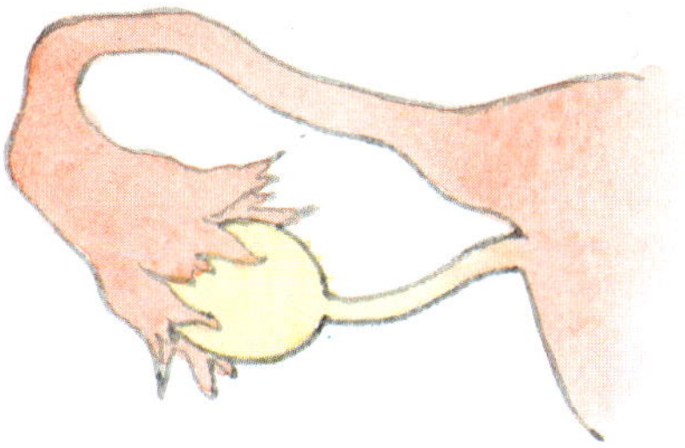

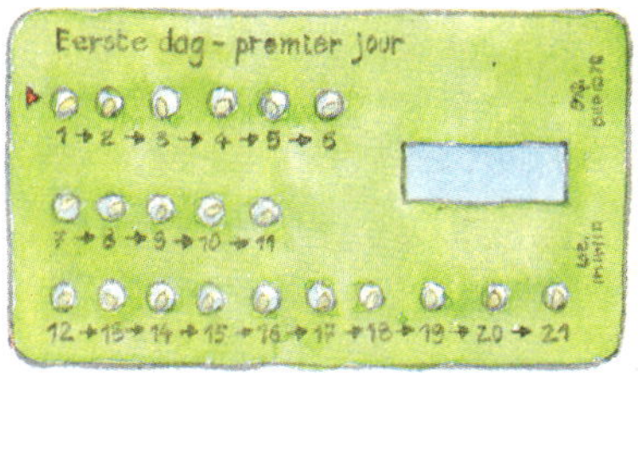

*The **Pill** either prevents eggs from ripening in the ovaries or it prevents the egg from embedding itself in the lining of the uterus.*

developed and has not, so far, proved to be very popular.

An alternative device is the collatex sponge. This is a soft, disposable foam sponge which contains spermicide. The woman inserts it into the vagina before sexual intercourse and it is left in for some time so that the sperm are killed. Like the cap and female condom, this is about 93% effective.

If, for any reason, a couple have made love without any protection, or, in very rare cases, when a condom has split, the woman can take a 'morning after' pill, which can be obtained from a doctor or family planning clinic. This pill contains high levels of progesterone and oestrogen, or just oestrogen, and it must be taken within 72 hours (three days) of making love.

When a couple have completed their family they may feel they are ready for sterilisation. Either the woman or the man can be sterilised. In women the Fallopian tubes are cut or tied off. In this way, eggs and sperm are prevented from meeting. In the man, the vas deferens are cut or tied off and the sperm do not leave the penis. Sterilisation is usually reversible in women but an operation to reverse the process for a man is not always successful.

• Can all women have babies?

Most women are able to become pregnant if they make love without contraception during ovulation. For some women who are trying to start a family, however, it can be very frustrating when they find out that they seem un-

The following problems may prevent pregnancy

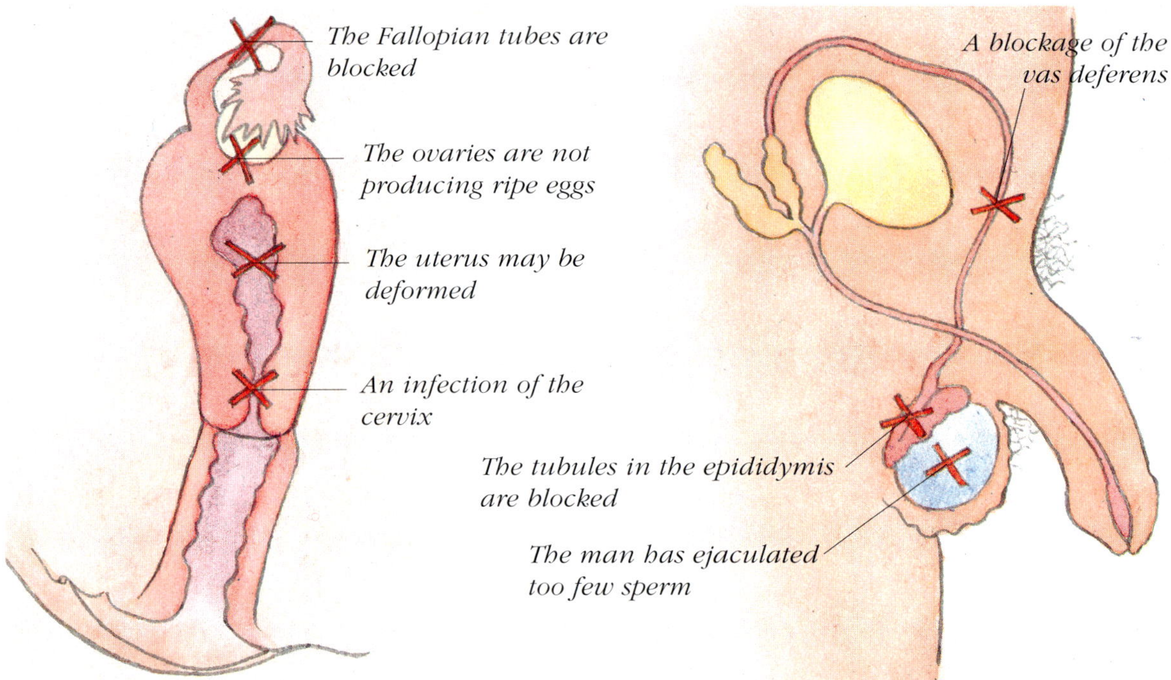

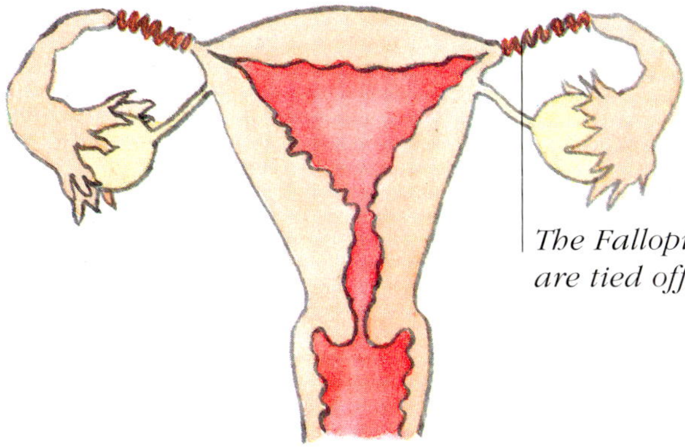

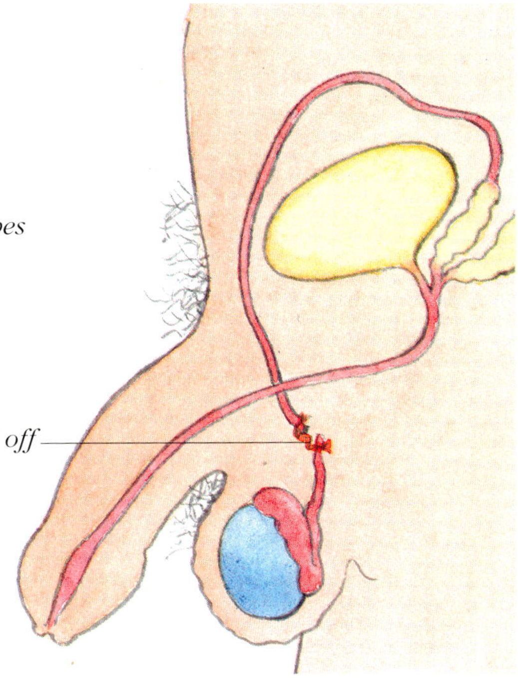

Sterilisation is a simple surgical operation that may be performed on either a man or a woman.

able to become pregnant.

In such cases, a doctor will examine the woman and her partner to find out what the problem is. It may be that the woman's Fallopian tubes are blocked or her ovaries may not be functioning correctly due to anaemia or a hormonal disease. She may have an infection in her uterus or vagina, or she may not have enough cervical mucus to help the sperm swim efficiently. All of these may be treated by either surgical intervention or medication.

Alternatively, the problem may lie with the man. He may not be able to keep an erection for long enough to enter the woman or his sperm cannot swim properly because they are not fully developed. It may be that there are not enough sperm being ejaculated. These problems can all be investigated and treated effectively.

For example, the man's sperm can be helped on their way by being introduced into the woman during ovulation using a syringe – this is called artificial insemination.

When the man's sperm are not mobile enough, the couple may use sperm which have been provided by a donor. In such cases the donor is another man, usually a stranger, who has ejaculated his sperm into a container and left it at a special clinic. Couples who use a donor's sperm are not told his name. If surgical intervention or treatment does not work, the couple may consider IVF (In Vitro Fertilisation). This is when an egg is removed from the woman and placed with the man's sperm in a test tube. If a sperm fertilises the egg, it is placed inside the woman's uterus.

When the baby, or babies if several eggs have been used, are born, they are referred to as 'test tube babies'.

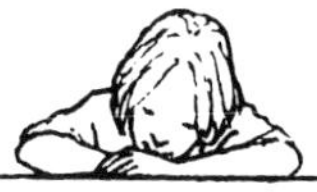

My aunt was three months pregnant when she lost her baby. I remember she was really upset about it. She had to go to the hospital for a D and C. My mother told me that stands for dilation and curetage. This is when the doctor cleans the inner surface of the womb.
When my aunt became pregnant nine months ago, everything was all right and she's just had a baby boy.

Sara, 11 years old

• Why do some women have miscarriages?

Sometimes pregnant women lose their babies while they are still forming. If so, it is usually during the first three months of pregnancy and often before the woman has realised that she is pregnant. There are several causes of miscarriage. The most common is when an egg has been fertilised by a damaged sperm. The embryo is imperfect and a miscarriage is nature's way of preventing the creation of a badly disabled child. Another cause may be an imbalance in the woman's hormones. Her hormone levels are not being controlled as they should be and the pregnancy is not able to continue.
Occasionally a woman's hormonal balance is disrupted by a severe shock or upset. This is relatively rare, however.
Sometimes a fertilised egg embeds itself in the lining of the Fallopian tube and grows there. An embryo growing here is very painful and it usually ends in a miscarriage. Another cause of miscarriage may be that the cervix has not stayed firmly closed.
This problem can be solved by a few stitches which hold the cervix closed until the baby is ready to be born.
A miscarriage may also be caused by the woman's immune system which reacts to the embryo as if it were a harmful invading micro-organism.

• What is a termination?

A termination is another word for an abortion.
This is when the woman or couple decide to end the pregnancy.
There may be many reasons for this decision, such as the age and or lifestyle of the woman, the probability of a badly deformed child, or rape. The girl or woman will ask a doctor to give his consent to an abortion.
If a young girl has become pregnant she may need her parents' consent and the doctor will recommend counselling to help her decide what to do. Provided that the decision is made early on in a pregnancy, a doctor can remove the embryo from the uterus while the woman is under general anaesthetic.

• Can a pregnant woman pass an infection to the foetus?

Pregnant women generally have excellent immune systems and they are ill less often than usual.
Doctors will often advise pregnant wo-

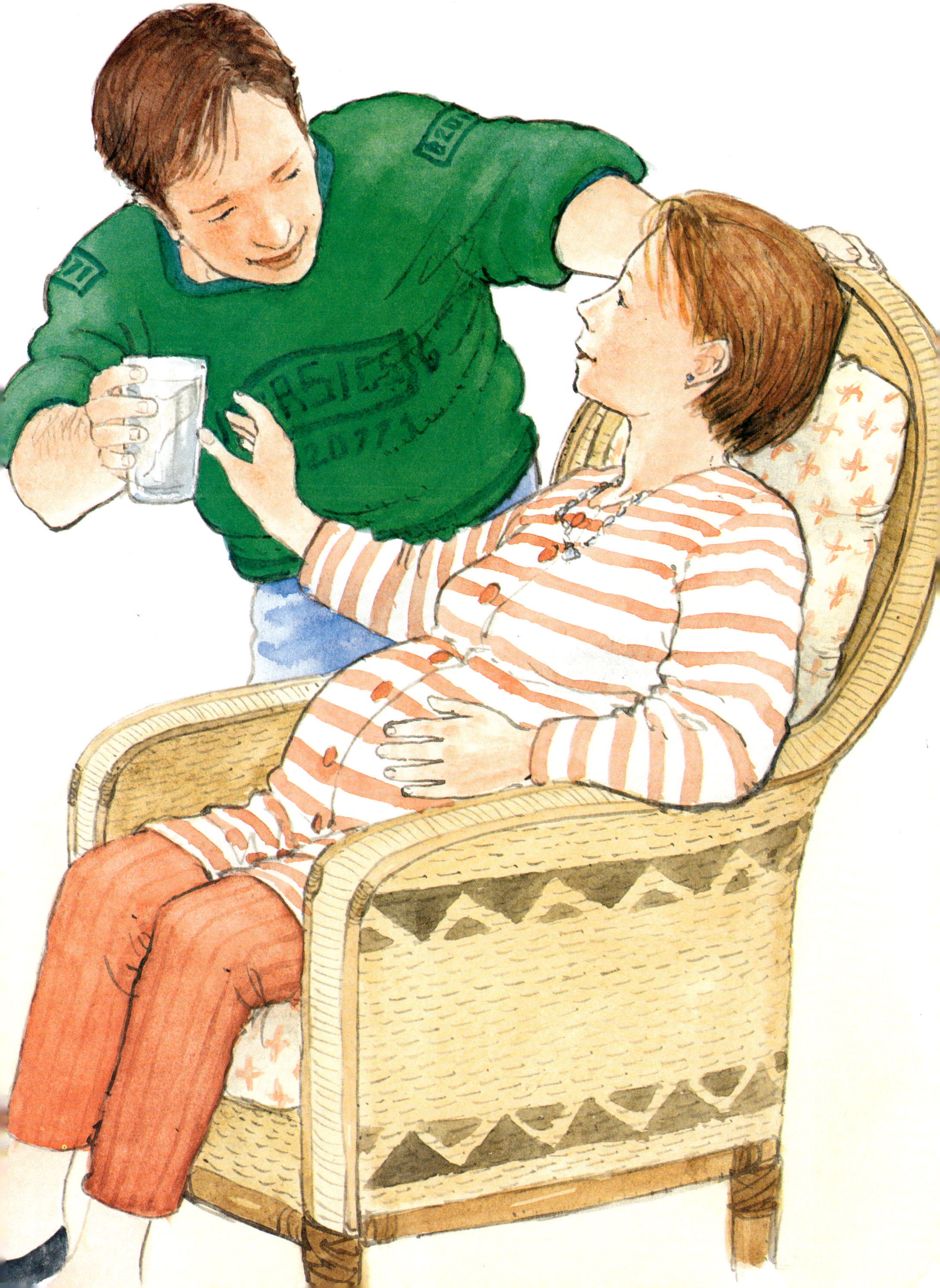

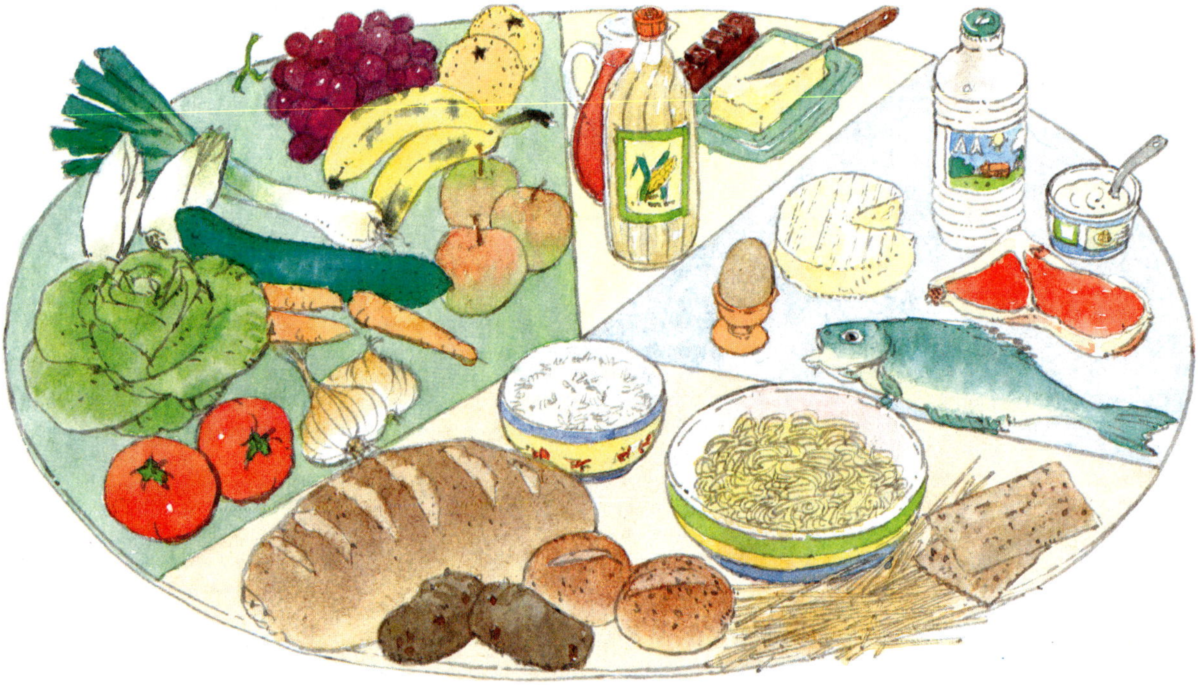

A healthy, balanced diet is very important during pregnancy.

men against taking medication during a pregnancy because they can be harmful to the foetus. Most women have a blood test before becoming pregnant. If the blood does not contain antibodies for rubella (German measles) the doctor will recommend that the woman is given a vaccination against the disease. Those women who have become pregnant without having had either the vaccination or the disease are warned to keep away from children (and in rare cases, adults) who are suffering from it. If a pregnant woman catches German measles her baby may be damaged and become blind, deaf or suffer from heart defects.

Pregnant women are also warned to keep away from dogs' and cats' faeces. These animals' droppings can contain the micro-organisms that cause toxoplasmosis. Uncooked meat, raw eggs and unwashed vegetables should also be avoided as they can carry the harmful micro-organisms too.

The micro-organisms are able to pass from the mother's blood to the foetus and affect its development. Babies are born with serious deformities.

Eating healthily

Pregnant women should avoid smoking and drinking alcohol as these can cause babies to be born prematurely. Such babies are usually smaller than average, too. Taking drugs is especially harmful because it can prevent the baby's limbs from forming properly. All pregnant women should drink plenty of water and eat healthily.

FROM EMBRYO TO BABY

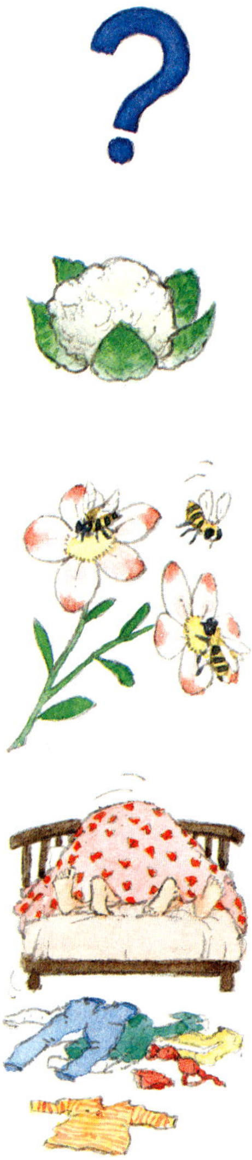

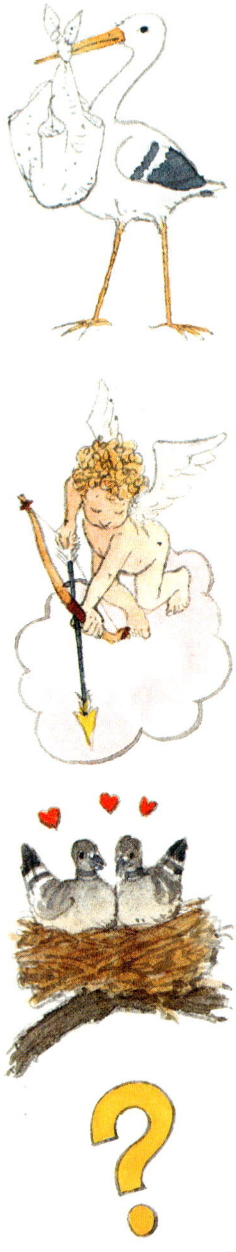

You have already discovered how the egg is fertilised and how it attaches itself to the lining of the uterus. The fertilised egg becomes a ball of cells which divide and divide. The ball of cells is referred to as an embryo. When the embryo is 12 weeks old it is about nine centimetres long. It looks human and it is called a foetus.

Pregnancy is an exciting time for the future parents. It is a time of wonder and joy. However, it can be uncomfortable for the woman, too. In fact the hormones produced by the woman's body at this time cause morning (or evening) sickness during the early weeks of a pregnancy. If all goes well, the foetus will develop inside the woman's uterus until, after nine months, the tiny embryo has become a fully formed baby and it is ready to be born.

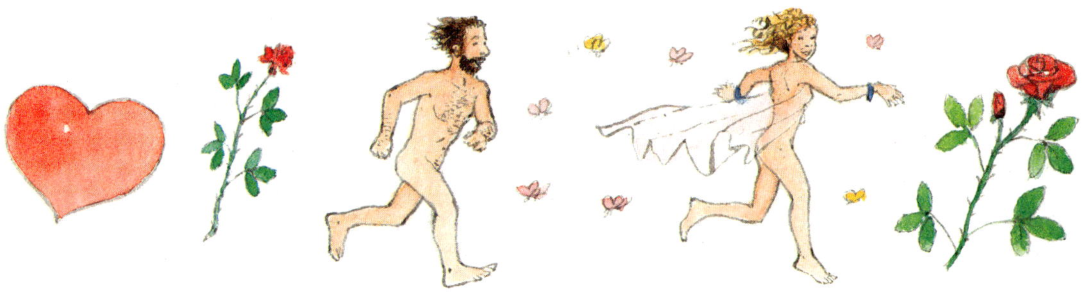

• How do cells become organs?

The 46 chromosomes in the embryo determine what will happen to the cells which are created by the process of division. Some of the cells will become the tissue of the umbilical cord which links the embryo to the uterus and the rest will go on to make up the baby's body. The chromosomes also decide which cells become the specialised cells that make up the different parts of the body.

A fertilised egg starts by dividing into two. The division of these two cells means there are four cells. The four cells divide into eight, the eight into 16, 16 into 32, and so on. Eventually the cells form groups which develop into a head, legs, arms, a heart etc.

The embryo in the uterus

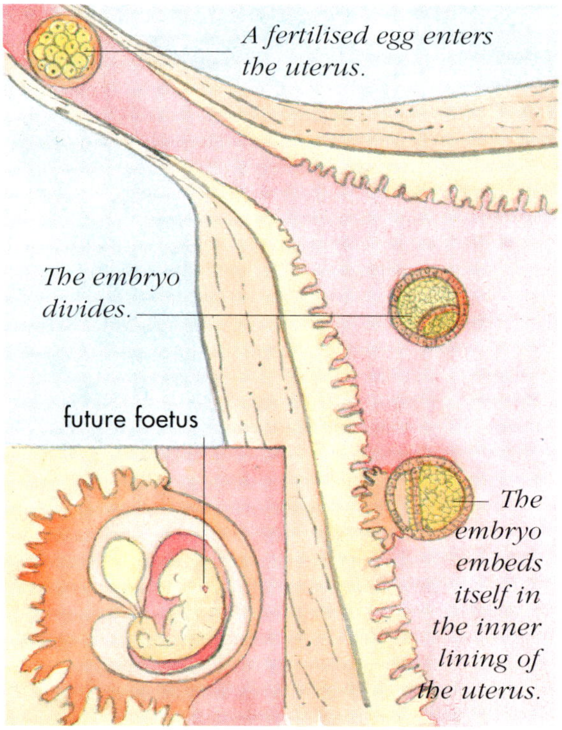

From embryo to baby.

By the end of the pregnancy the baby weighs 10 times its weight as at the middle of the pregnancy.

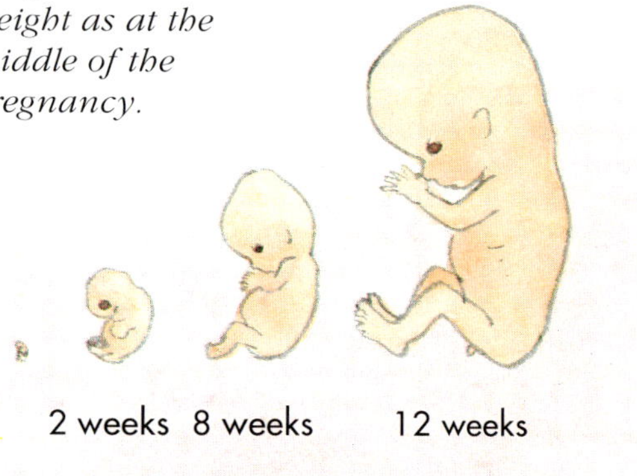

• What are the stages in the development of the foetus?

A foetus develops quickly. By the fifth week the embryo is about 2 mm long. The spine is just about visible.

During the sixth week, however, the head is forming and then the chest and stomach develop. In the seventh week the embryo develops arms and legs. These are soon followed by the neck, eyes, ears, blood vessels and intestines. Its heart is pumping blood round the body and the liver and kidneys are formed. The embryo is just over 1 cm long.

During the eighth week the vital internal organs grow and develop. The embryo's head is large compared to the rest of its body and its eyes, nostrils and ears are showing.

By week 20, the foetus is about 10 inches (25 cm) long. It has downy hair on its body and it is able to kick and rotate. After 24 weeks, the foetus opens its eyes when it is awake.

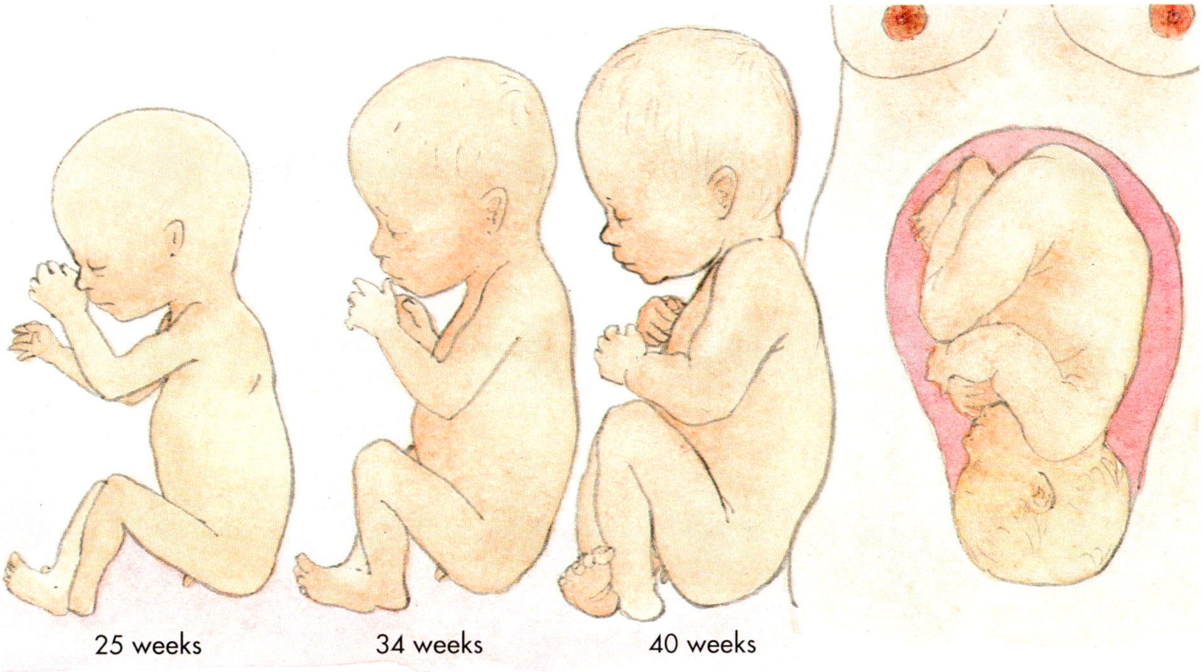

It could survive for a short while if it were born but it is during the last three months that it grows and develops to its proper size. When it is born a baby weighs on average between two and three kilos (about 2 1/2 lb).

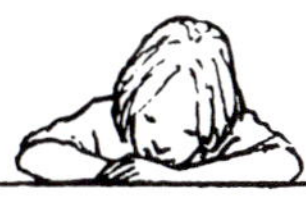

My mum has been pregnant for five months and the last time she went to the doctor I went with her. The doctor put some clear gel on her stomach and then he put a sort of camera on it. We saw the baby on a screen. At first I couldn't see where its head was, but the doctor showed us the different parts of the baby. Then I could see its head, arms and legs. I could even see its fingers. The doctor said he could tell us if it would be a boy or a girl. He asked Mummy if she wanted to know, but she said she wanted it to be a surprise.

Zoe, 8 years old

• Do babies breathe inside the uterus?

Humans need to take in oxygen and breathe out carbon dioxide in order to live. A baby cannot breathe when it is in the uterus because it surrounded by a fluid called amniotic fluid. Furthermore, for most of the time that it is in the uterus, the baby's lungs are not fully developed.
However, the baby still needs to take in oxygen and get rid of carbon dioxide. It does this via the placenta.
The placenta is a dish-shaped organ that is made up partly of the mother's tissues and partly from those of the baby.
The baby's blood is carried to and from the placenta in the blood vessels of the umbilical cord.
In the placenta the mother's blood vessels pass close to those of her baby. Oxygen from the mother's blood passes into her baby's blood and carbon dioxide from the baby's blood passes

Getting into practice?

Although a baby cannot breathe in air inside the uterus, its lungs and chest appear to be moving. Is it practising for later?
Gulping amniotic fluid may also cause the baby to hiccough occasionally.

into that of the mother.
Food is also passed to the baby in this way and the baby uses the placenta to get rid of waste materials.
This is happening all the time that the baby is in the uterus. At birth, the baby takes its first breath and the umbilical cord is no longer necessary. It is cut and clamped off.

• Do babies drink the amniotic fluid?

Yes, babies drink the amniotic fluid and also urinate into it. This seems like an unhygienic situation but in fact the amniotic fluid is renewed 10 to 20 times every 24 hours. This amounts to 15 litres a day.
The renewal of amniotic fluid helps to get rid of a baby's waste products and this is vital to its health.
As well as drinking the amniotic fluid, the baby absorbs some of it through its skin. The fluid enters the bloodstream and is passed into the mother's blood via the placenta.

• Why should pregnant women drink lots of water?

When a woman is pregnant her body needs more water, although not in excessive quantities. The amniotic fluid that is filtered into the uterus is mostly made up of water.

• How are babies protected from bumps and jolts?

A baby will not usually feel anything if the mother knocks against something hard.
This is because it is cushioned by the amniotic fluid which is contained in a thin membrane called the amniotic sac.
When the woman bumps her stomach against something, the shock is absorbed by the fluid.
Imagine if you were in a swimming pool and someone jumped in beside you.
This is the sort of effect felt by the baby inside the amniotic sac.
The fluid around the baby also helps to keep its body temperature constant.

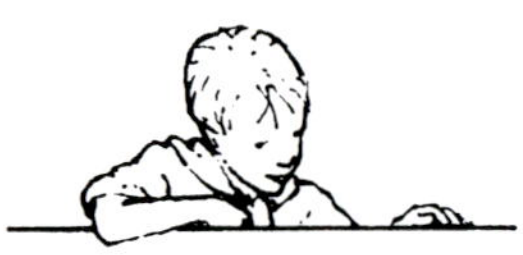

My brother's wife is pregnant. She is huge. She looks as if she has swallowed a balloon. I asked my brother if he still made love to her. He said he did, but I wonder how they manage with her big stomach.

Jonathan, 14 years old

• Can babies become ill in the uterus?

The placenta acts as a barrier that prevents micro-organisms, such as bacteria, or viruses, passing from the mother to the baby. Certain diseases can pass into the baby's blood, such as rubella and toxoplasmosis.
Some harmful substances, for example, alcohol or drugs, can also pass across. It is the mother's responsibility to be aware of this and to reduce her intake of alcohol, drugs and cigarette smoke or, better still, to avoid them altogether.

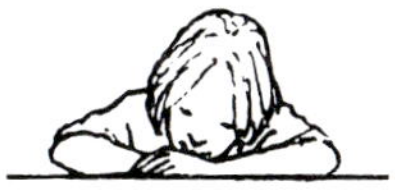

My elder sister is pregnant. When I went to stay at her house she was having morning sickness. One day I saw her eating cracker biscuits in bed before she got up. She told me it made her feel less ill.

Alison, 16 years old

• Do babies dream?

Yes, a baby can dream, but its dreams are different from ours. It has no idea of what the world is like nor of what is happening around it. The dreams of a baby are unstructured. They are short, vague sensations of noises and motions that have entered its tiny environment. The dreams consist of remembering any event that has occured, such as sucking its thumb, touching its umbili-

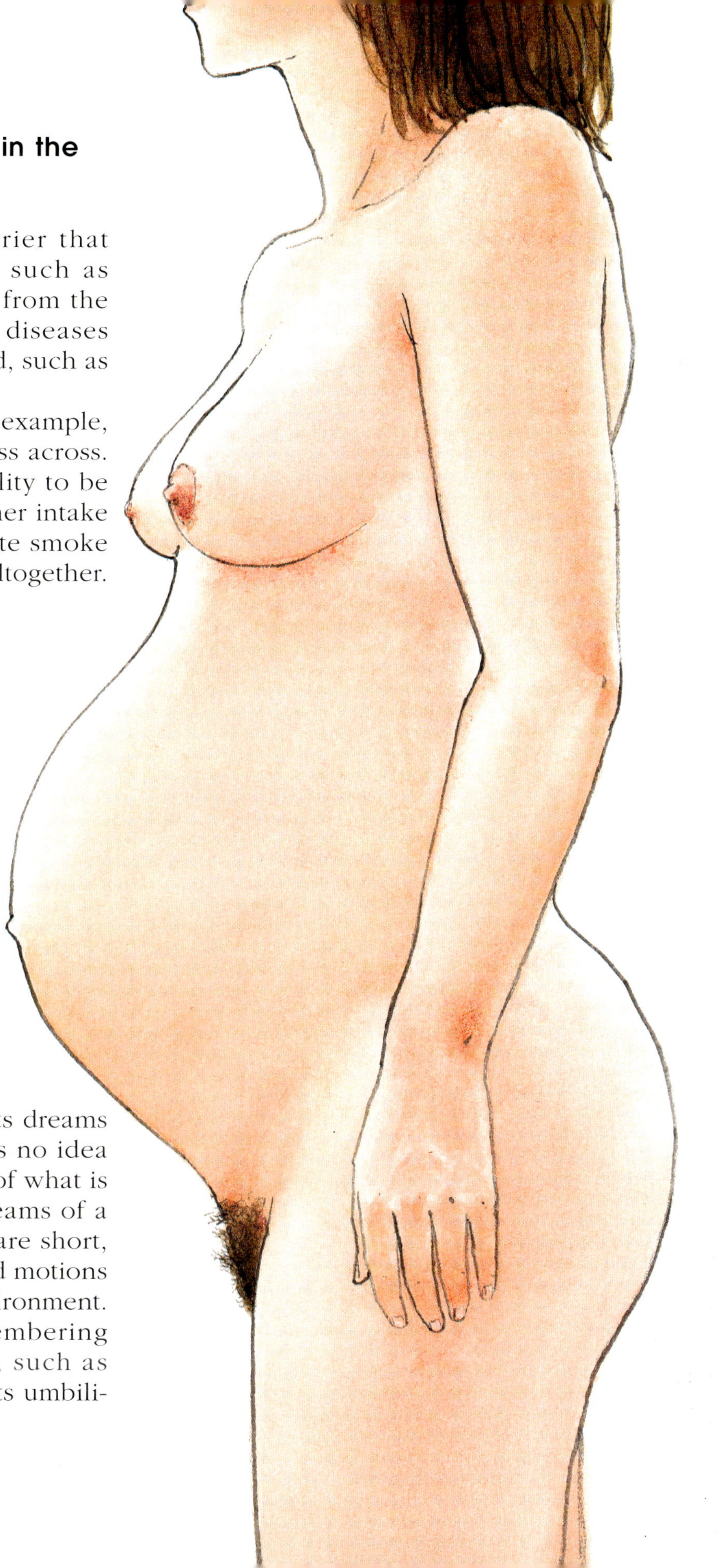

cal cord with its hands, its mother's voice, pleasant sounds or any movement it has felt through the vibrations of the amniotic fluid.
A baby can also feel distressed or content. These feelings would probably enter its dreams too.

• Is it possible to communicate with a baby?

During the second half of a pregnancy the baby is aware of certain sounds. Sounds such as those produced by the circulation of its mother's blood or her heartbeat assure and calm the baby. The gurgling sounds of the woman's digestive system are also familiar.
Sounds from outside the body can also be heard, for example, harsh, loud music or the slam of a door.
Often these sounds appear to disturb the baby. It reacts by waving its limbs about. These movements can often be felt by the mother who says that her baby is 'kicking'.
Some parents like to play gentle music to soothe their baby during the last few months of pregnancy. Once the baby is born, it seems that the same music can soothe the infant when it is restless.
Other mothers sing lullabies to their baby before it is born for the same reason.
If you put your mouth close to a pregnant woman's stomach and talk to the baby it can hear you.
It learns to recognise the voices that are most familiar and that it hears often.
If the mother puts her hand on her stomach, the baby can be seen moving towards the hand. It is, therefore, possible to play with it before it is born!

When Mummy jumps I shake my arms in sympathy

When a pregnant woman jumps or starts with shock, her baby waves its arms and legs. When the pregnant woman is startled, a certain hormone is produced in her bloodstream and her heartbeat accelerates. These two signals are intercepted by the baby and it reacts by agitating its limbs.

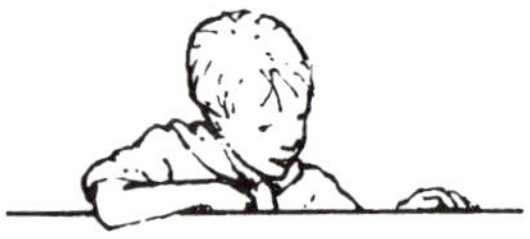

Mummy is going to have a baby soon. Sometimes she lets me put my hand on her tummy and I can feel the baby kicking. I asked Mummy if it hurt her and she said it didn't. She likes feeling the baby move about. I don't think it should kick me though.

James, 6 years old

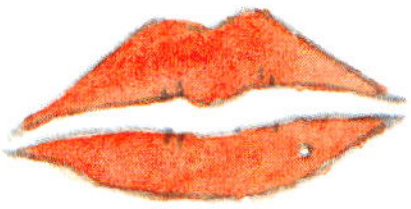
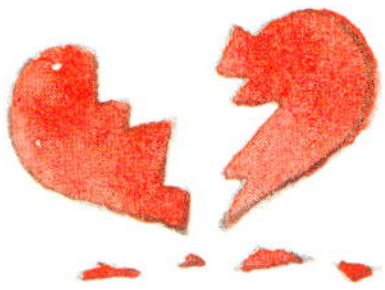
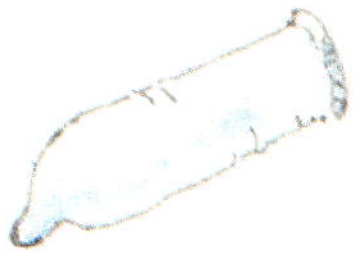
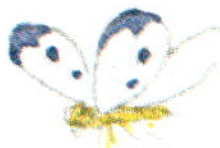
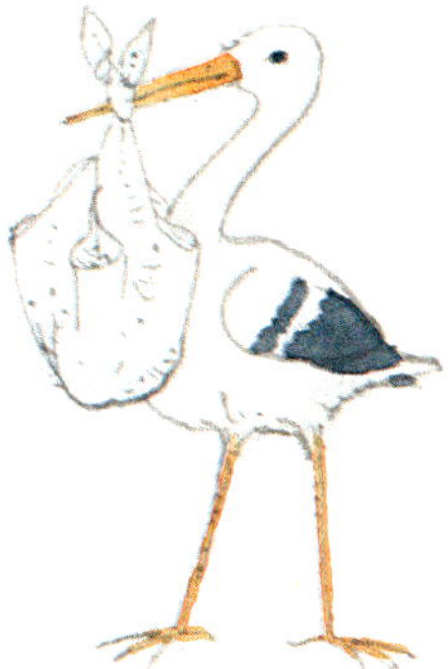

BIRTH

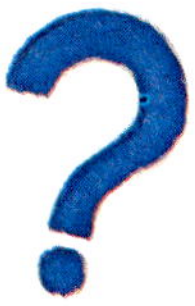

In the past, it was common for women to give birth at home. Nowadays most women are expected to give birth in hospital, especially if it is their first baby.

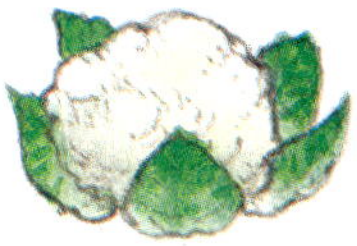
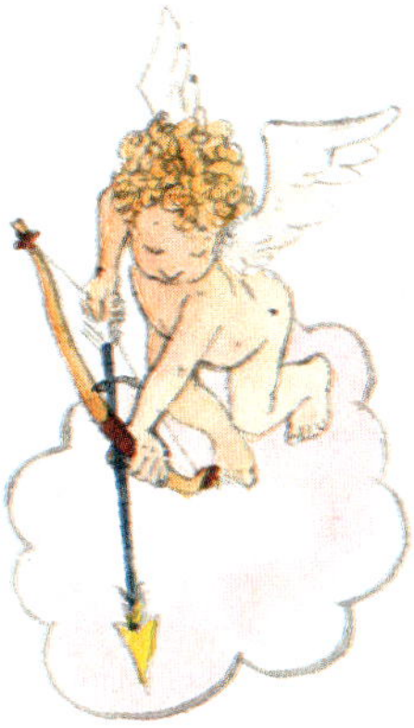

Giving birth at home, however, is still preferred by some women who feel uncomfortable in the unfamiliar surroundings of a hospital. They feel more relaxed at home where they are surrounded by their own possessions and can easily take warm baths to ease the pain.

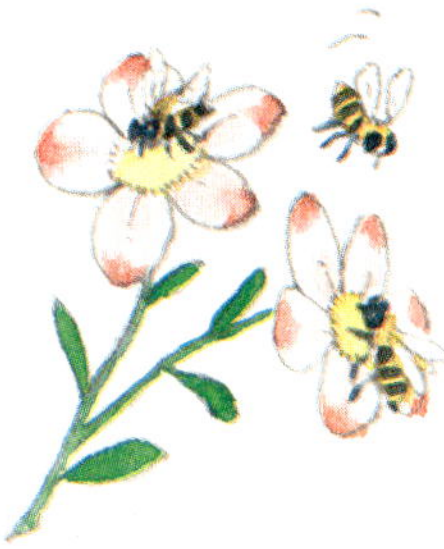
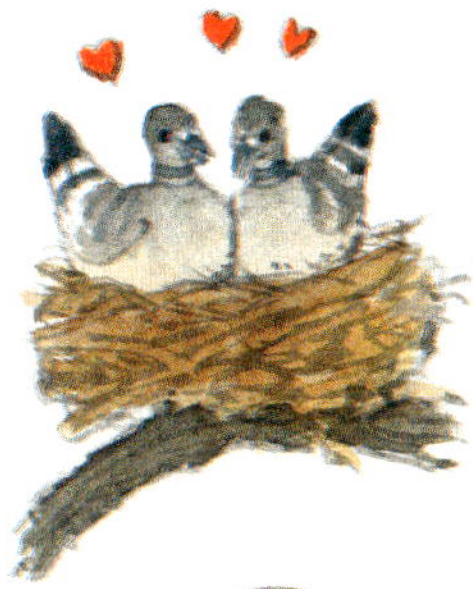

Women who give birth in hospital often feel safer there because they know a doctor is nearby in case of complications. If it is their first baby they may feel nervous and it is reassuring for them to see other women who are in the same condition.

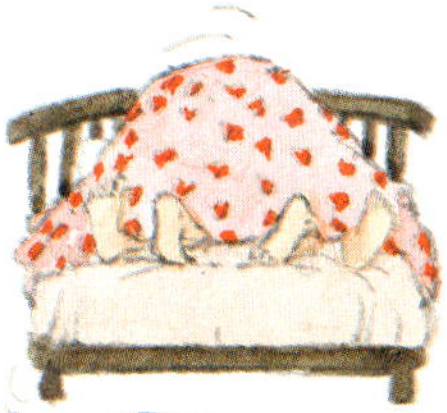
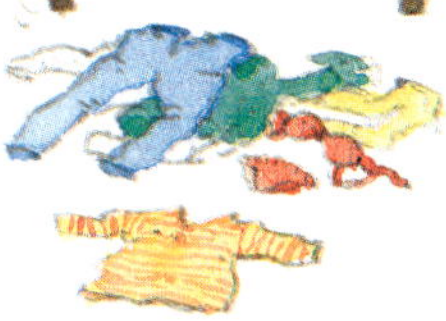
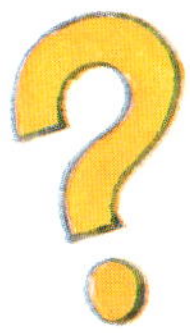

In the old days, giving birth was a private matter that concerned only the mother and the doctor or midwife. Fathers waited outside the room or the house until the baby was born. The children of the family were told that their mother had broken a leg or an arm. The situation today is quite different. Fathers and family are encouraged to support the mother when she gives birth. The following pages will explain how a baby is born.

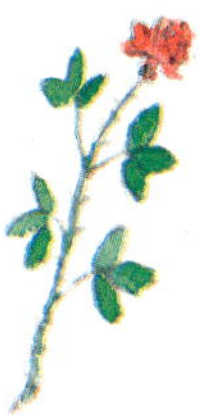
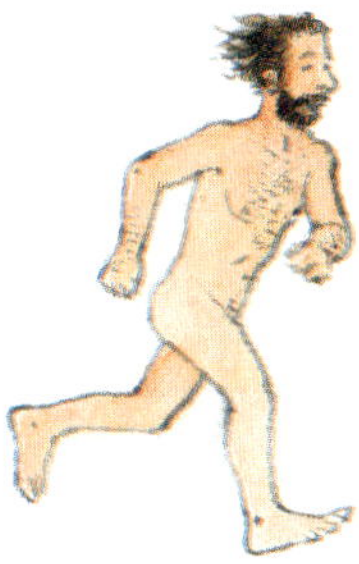
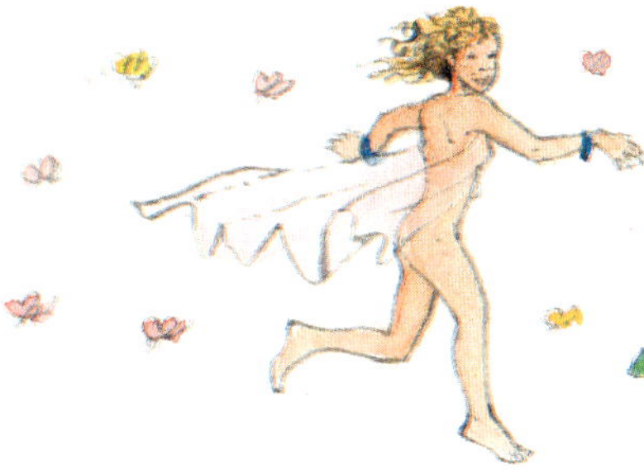
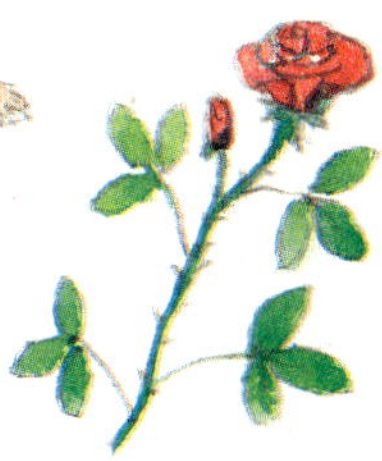

• Why do pregnant women go to antenatal classes?

Bringing a baby into the world requires great physical effort. To help prepare for giving birth many expectant mothers attend antenatal classes.

When a woman gives birth, her uterus contracts. This is known as being in labour and, although the contractions do not harm the baby, they are painful for the mother and they can continue for several hours.

Antenatal classes are given by qualified midwives who tell expectant mothers what to expect during labour and what will happen to their bodies when they give birth. They also teach breathing exercises to help them relax and to cope with the stress of labour.

Sometimes being pregnant and having the added weight of the baby inside their uterus causes women to suffer from backache. Antenatal classes can help women with their posture and teach them specially devised, gentle exercises to help them keep fit.

Good posture and overall fitness can prevent or relieve backache. Regular swimming is another good way for pregnant women to keep fit.

During antenatal classes pregnant women learn how to recognise when they are in labour and how to push when it comes to helping the baby out of the body.

Fathers-to-be are encouraged to attend the classes to learn how to help and support the woman during labour.

Many women enjoy going to antenatal classes because they meet other pregnant women and share ideas.

From a pear to a balloon

During pregnancy, the shape of the uterus changes. It starts off as a small pear-shaped organ and becomes as large as a balloon. At the end of the pregnancy, the uterus takes up most of the space inside a woman's abdomen.

• In what position does the baby lie in the uterus?

At the beginning of a pregnancy the foetus is so small that the woman cannot feel it moving. From the fourth month onwards, however, she begins to feel it moving. The baby is floating like an astronaut in the amniotic fluid inside the uterus and because it has plenty of space it is able to move freely and even do somersaults.

Towards the end of the pregnancy, the baby has grown so much that there is not much room for it to move. After 36 weeks (eight months), the baby positions itself head down in the uterus. This is the best position for it to leave the mother's body. The baby's head is larger than any other part of its body and once it has passed out of the vagina, the rest of the body slips through relatively easily. Sometimes the baby positions itself the other way up and tries to come out bottom first – this is called a breech birth. A breech birth is difficult because the baby's head cannot lead the way out.

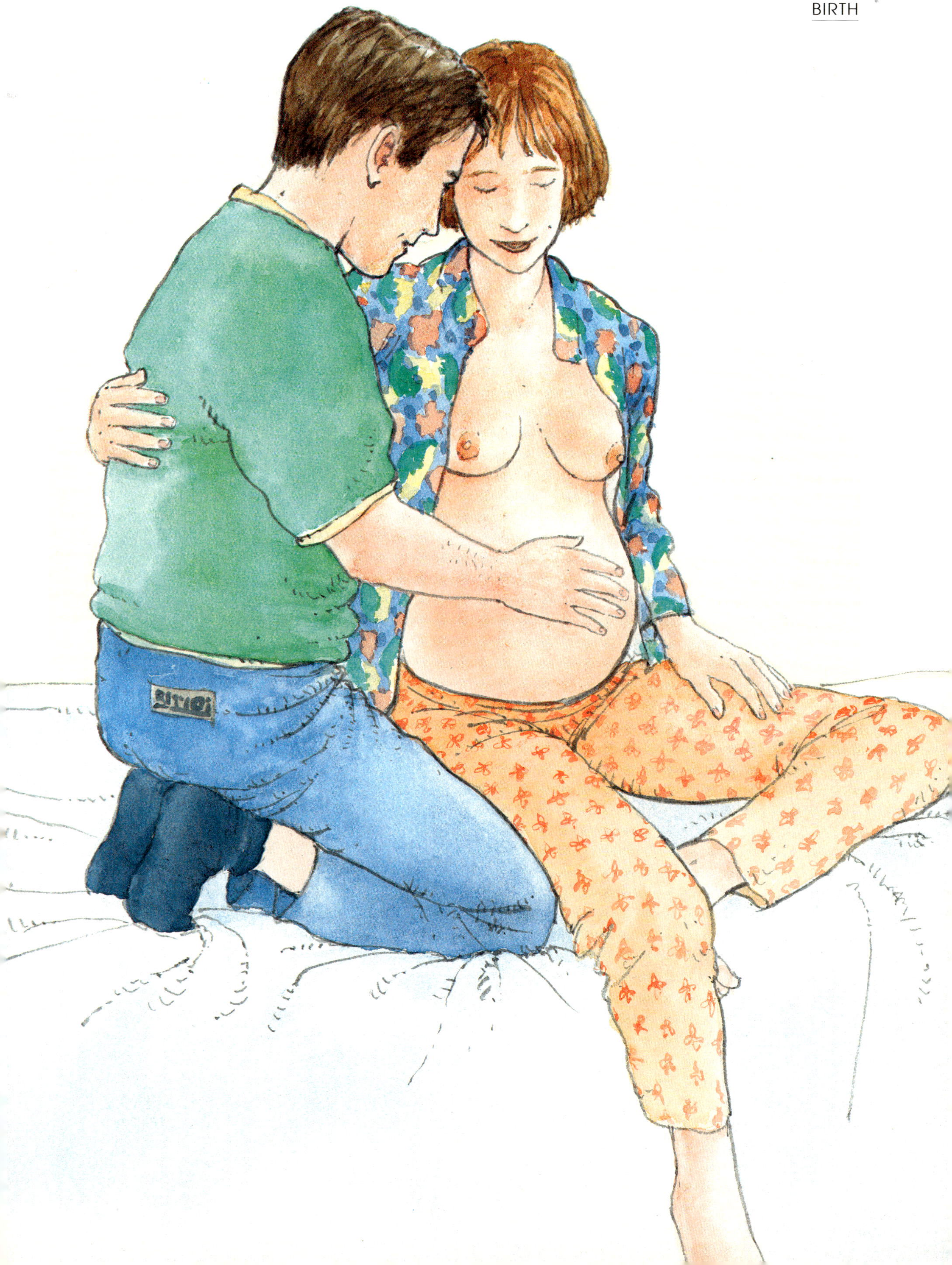

• When is the baby ready to be born?

A baby is ready to leave the uterus about 40 weeks after the egg was fertilised by the sperm.
Some babies leave the uterus a few weeks early while others, usually those in a first pregnancy, are often late.
Babies that are born before the end of nine months are called premature babies. If they are very early or particularly small they may need to be placed in an incubator where they are kept warm and free of germs. The temperature inside an incubator is carefully monitored so that it stays the same.
If a baby is severely premature, its organs will probably be underdeveloped and the infant will need oxygen via a tube into its nose to help it to breathe, and liquid food through a drip connected to its blood stream.
Babies that stay in the uterus after the end of nine months may need to be encouraged to come out. The doctor will give certain drugs to the mother which cause labour to start. This is known as inducing labour.

What is a 'viable' foetus?

A 'viable' foetus is one that has spent seven months in the uterus. If the baby were born it might survive if it had very special care and attention.
A baby born after only seven months in the uterus is very small and weighs less than one kilo.

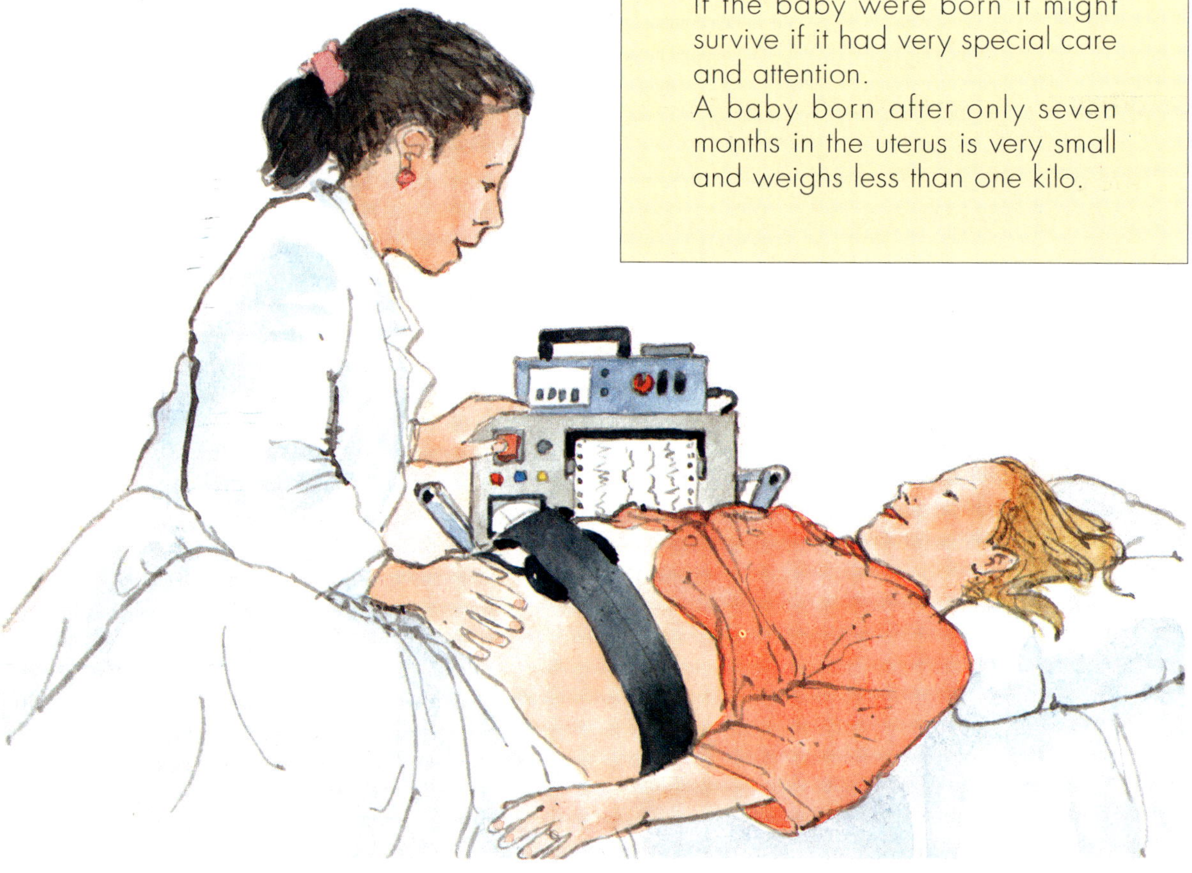

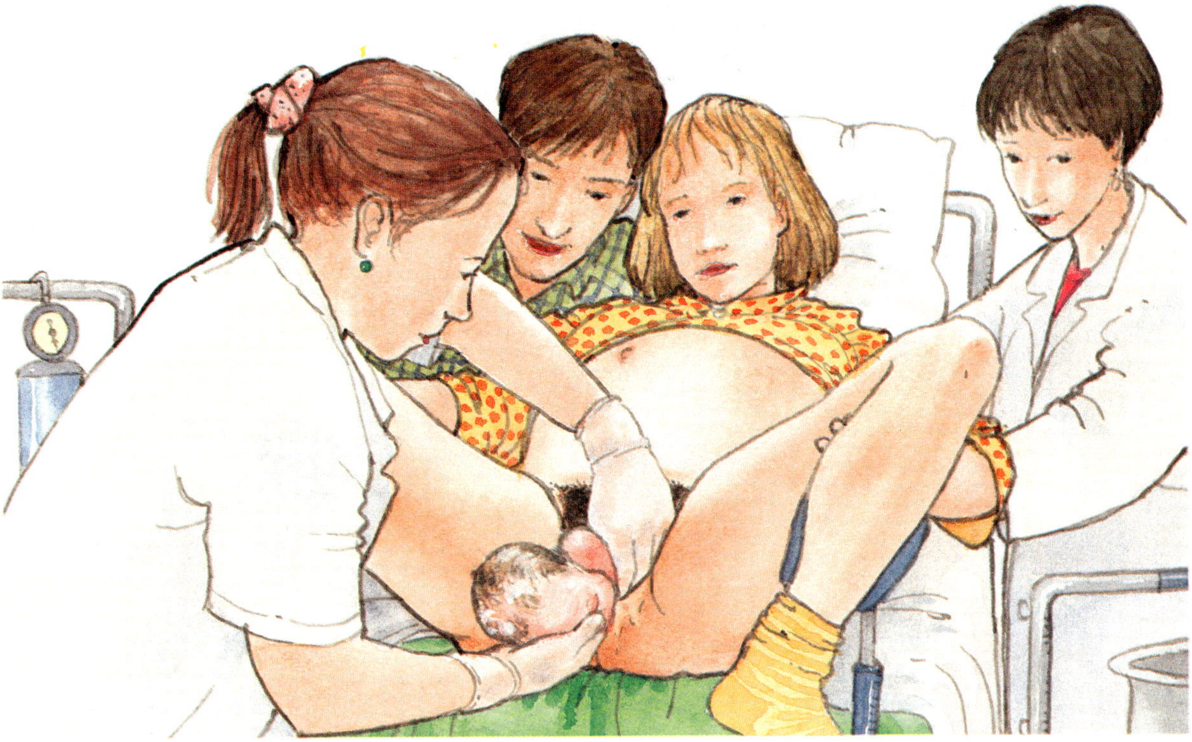

• What happens during labour?

At the end of nine months in the uterus, labour is stimulated by the production of certain hormones and the pressure of the baby's head on the cervix.

The baby is ready to be born and the mother is, by this time, ready to give birth. The mother will probably have been uncomfortable and had restless nights during the last few weeks because the baby is heavy and its size means it is pressing on her internal organs. When the baby turns upside down, the doctor or midwife is able to tell its position by feeling the mother's abdomen. They are able to warn the mother that it will soon be time to give birth.

A woman will feel irregular contractions before labour really starts. When the contractions become painful and regular, the woman knows labour has started. The uterus contracting in this way helps to push the baby downwards towards the cervix. A plug of mucus, which has been keeping the cervix moist and lubricated, breaks away as the cervix starts to open (dilate).

The pressure of the baby's head on the amniotic sac causes it to break and the amniotic fluid flows out. This is known as 'breaking the waters' and it can be a sign that the baby is about to be born. The breathing exercises that the mother has learnt in antenatal classes will help her to cope with the pain of contractions. If the mother and her partner have arranged a hospital birth, this is when they should go to the hospital. Once there, the doctor or midwife will

A mother-to-be knows her baby is about to be born when:

- the plug of mucus breaks away from the cervix and passes out of the vagina;
- the contractions occur regularly at five to seven minutes apart;
- her waters break;
- for about 10% of women, the first sign that they are near to giving birth is the sight of water trickling down their legs.

measure the dilation (opening) of the cervix. When the cervix is fully ten centimetres across, it is fully dilated and the nature of the contractions change. They make the woman feel that she must push downwards to help the baby out.

With each contraction and push, the baby starts to leave the uterus and move through the vagina. The vagina stretches to allow room for the baby's head to pass. Once the baby's head reaches the opening of the vagina, its head rotates to the side and it is pushed out. The doctor or midwife help the rest of the body out.

The doctor or the midwife makes sure that the baby is breathing properly, before cutting the umbilical cord. This is completely painless for both the mother and the baby.

Labour is a painful process but once the mother is able to see and hold her baby she soon forgets her discomfort.

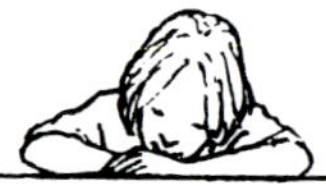

Mummy told me that giving birth to my brother was easier than when she had me. I was her first baby. The doctor said that the second birth is often easier and quicker than the first. The passages were stretched the first time and they didn't shrink back to the size they had been. So, I led the way for my baby brother.

Astrid, 12 years old

• How are twins born?

Twins are born just like other babies. They leave the uterus one at a time. It would be impossible for both to be born at once because the opening is too small. So one twin is always slightly older than the other.

Twins are usually smaller than other babies, but this is not because they are premature.

Nowadays an expectant mother is told quite early on in the pregnancy whether she is going to have twins. She will have time, therefore, to buy sufficient clothes, cots, bottles, and to choose two sets of names.

• Is it possible to have a painless labour?

If women find they are unable to cope with the pain of labour they may ask a doctor to give them an epidural.

This is a type of anaesthetic which is given to a woman via a narrow tube

and a needle that is inserted at the base of the spine.
The lower half of the woman's body becomes numb and she is unable to feel any pain when she gives birth.

• What happens during a home birth?

Providing there are no medical complications, there is no reason why women should not give birth at home.
Some women prefer to give birth at home where they feel more at ease with the familiar environment. Home births are attended by two midwives or a midwife and doctor.
The midwives will have had plenty of experience of home births and be able to recognise any signs of risk to mother and/or baby.
If a midwife detects a possible complication she will advise that the pregnant woman be taken to hospital where there are doctors and special equipment on hand.
When a woman is planning to give birth at home, the midwife will make sure that she has a bed on which to give birth, hot water, soap and basins or a bath for washing herself and the baby, as well as all the necessary towels.

• What does the baby feel during birth?

No one can remember what it is like being born, but it is almost certainly not a very pleasant experience.
The baby has been pushed and squashed out of its mother's warm body and

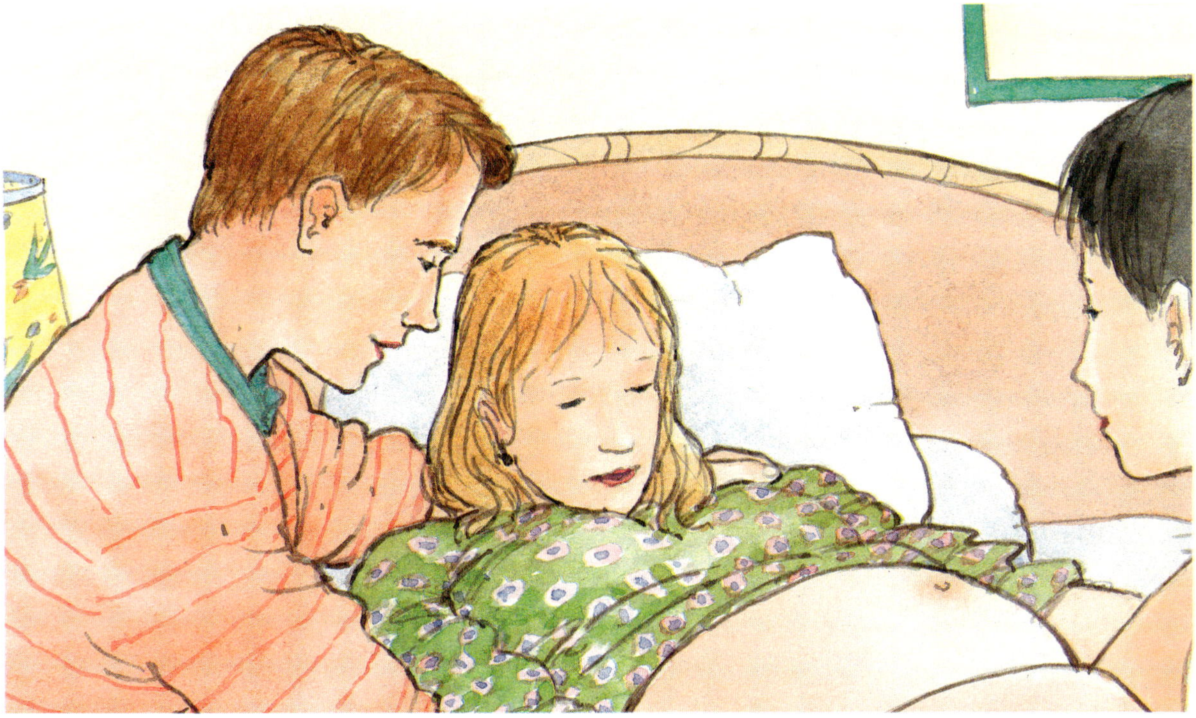

it is probably feeling tired and a bit crushed. Suddenly it is surrounded by air, light and lots of new noises. The baby may start to cry and often only a cuddle from its mother will comfort it. Sometimes this is when the baby will get its first suck on its mother's breast if it is hungry.
Later, after it has been washed, dried and dressed, the baby will feel more at ease. When it is returned to its mother for a cuddle it will be content. It will soon forget the unpleasant moments which accompanied its birth.
If it could talk, a baby would tell you that being born is not a nice experience, but it does not have any say in the matter.

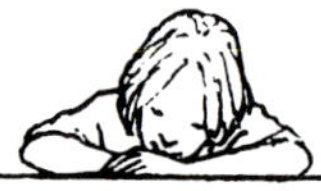

I was really surprised when I saw my little brother for the first time. He had just been born and he had a big bump on his head. I thought that someone must have dropped him. I asked Mummy and she told me that the birth had not been easy. The doctor had used a suction cup to help get my brother out of her tummy. After a few weeks the bump on his head had disappeared.

Leila, 7 years old

• What does a baby look like when it is born?

When a baby comes out of the vagina it may not look very pretty. A baby is usually covered with a whitish grease and smears of blood.
Its exit from the dark, warm uterus and entry into a cool, well-lit room can make it cry.
The mother is encouraged to hold her baby straight away.
She may want to place the naked baby on her bare stomach for a while.
This contact is called 'bonding'. It is supposed to make the baby feel close to its mother and more content.
Afterwards, the baby is washed and blobs of mucus are removed from its nostrils, mouth and ears.
The baby is dressed in its new clothes and it looks much better.

I am not very beautiful

During the last stage of labour when the baby is being pushed out of the vagina, it may not be able to breathe oxygen for a short while. This makes it look blue.
The baby's nose is often squashed and its eyelids can be swollen. The pressure of the birthing process will sometimes have pushed its facial bones out of place and its face may look slightly lopsided. Its genitals and breasts may also be slightly swollen after the birth. Many newborn babies have tiny white spots on their bodies. These are caused by sebum gathering in the sebaceous glands.
All of these symptoms disappear after a few hours.

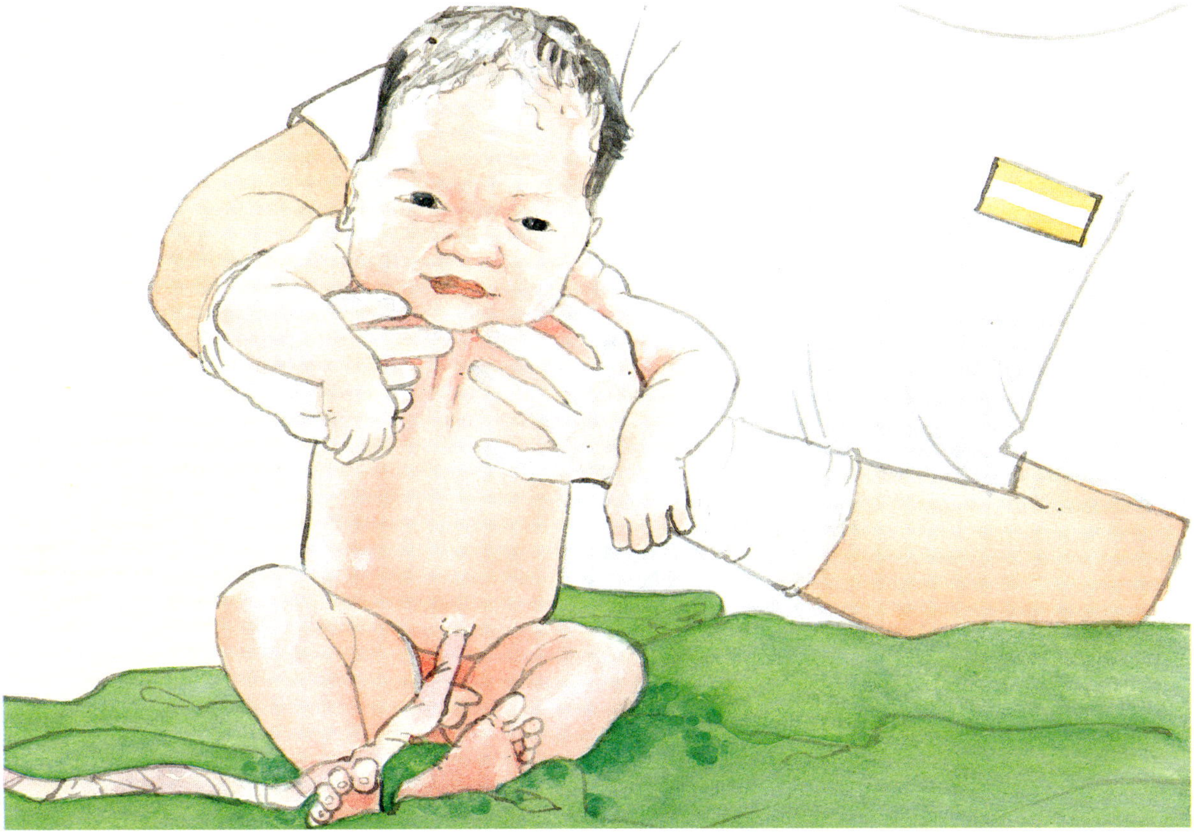

• Why do babies cry when they are born?

While the baby has been inside its mother's uterus, it has not needed to breathe air in and out. It has used oxygen from its mother's blood via the umbilical cord and the placenta. In fact, the baby has not been able to breathe because it has been surrounded by amniotic fluid. The fluid enters the baby's mouth when it is open and some of it is swallowed.

When the baby is born it is encouraged to breathe. If necessary, the doctor or midwife will remove mucus from the baby's mouth or throat. The action of crying will cause a newborn infant to draw breath in automatically.

• What happens to the placenta?

After the baby has been born, the placenta is no longer needed.

Further contractions of the uterus cause the placenta to detach itself from the wall. The contractions continue until the placenta has been pushed out of the vagina.

The mother may help by pushing in the same manner that helped the baby to be born.

The umbilical cord will have already been cut and clamped off.

A doctor or midwife will check the cord and placenta to make sure that there is nothing left behind in the mother's uterus.

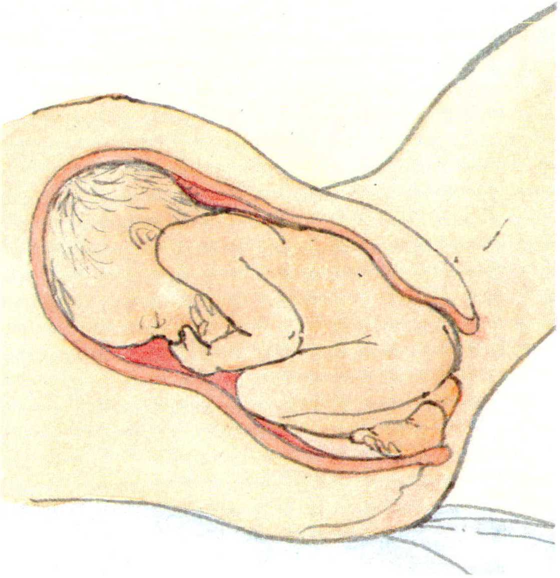

The baby tries to come out bottom first in a breech birth

• What happens during a breech birth?

A breech birth is when the baby comes out feet or bottom first. This type of birth can take more time than a normal delivery because the pressure of the baby's feet or bottom on the cervix is far less than that exerted by the head. This means that the cervix takes longer to dilate. Once the lower half of the baby has appeared in the vagina it is important that the baby's head follows quickly. If there is a risk that the delay will cause the baby to be deprived of oxygen, however, the doctor will resort to another method of delivery.

• What is a Caesarian section?

A Caesarian section is when a cut is made in the mother's abdomen and uterus, and the baby is taken out.
A Caesarian may be necessary if the mother has a small pelvis or if the baby is too big to pass out of the vagina. It may be that the placenta is blocking the cervix or there may be other complications which mean that the baby must be delivered rapidly.

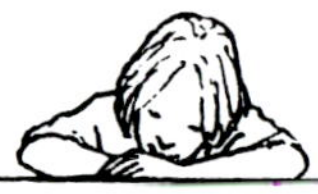

My best friend has got a new baby sister. Her mother had a narrow pelvis and the doctor performed a Caesarian section under local anaesthetic.
'Was she able to watch the whole operation?' I asked, horrified.
Lisa said no. She added that the doctor had hung a sort of screen over her mother's stomach so that she could not see what was happening. As soon as the baby was taken out, the doctor held it up for her mother to see.

Debbie, 12 years old

• Is a Caesarian section painful?

A Caesarian section is a painless process because the mother will have been given an anaesthetic beforehand. Women under general anaesthetic are unconscious when the Caesarian takes place. After the operation they wake up to find the baby beside them in a cot. Doctors will usually give a local anaesthetic, however, which allows the woman to follow the birth.
Her abdomen is numb and she does not feel any pain.

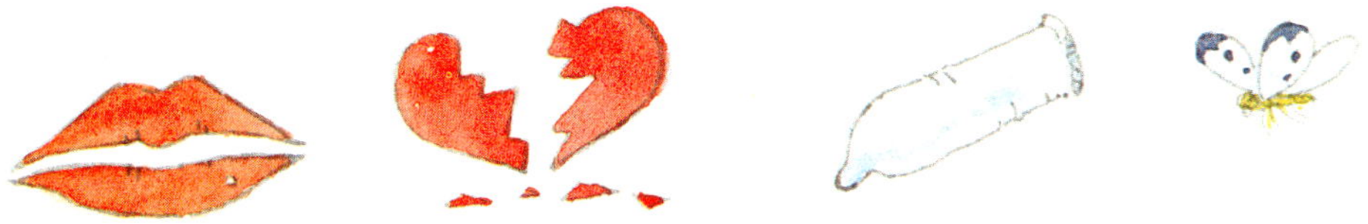

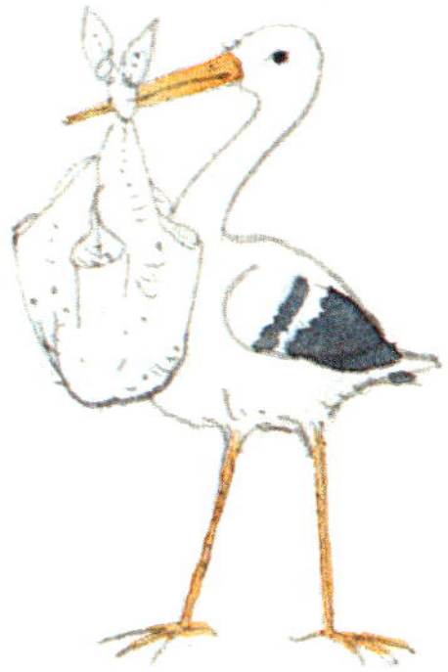

AFTER THE BIRTH

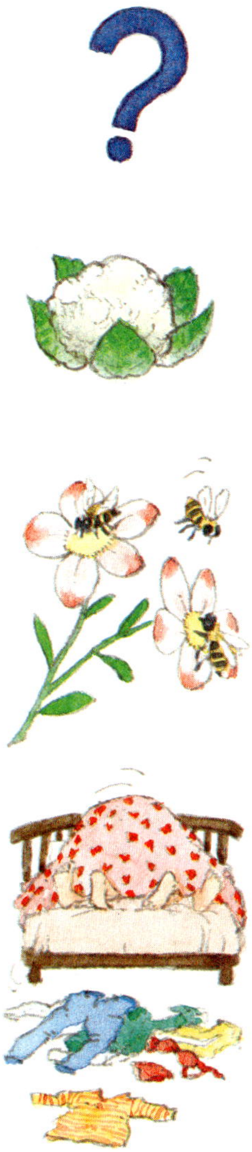

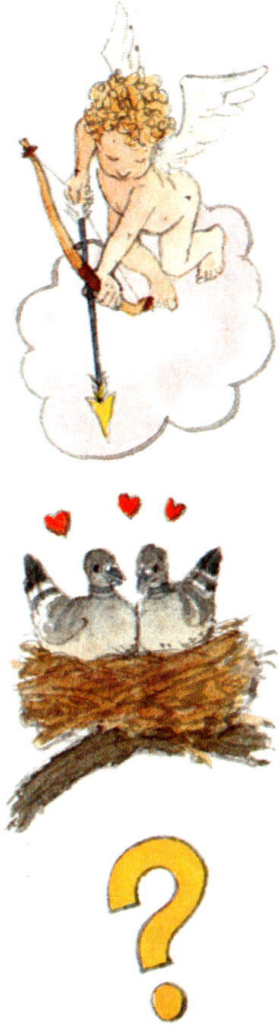

The first contact between a newborn baby and its parents is an extraordinary event. The baby is particularly alert during the first hour after being born. It recognises its mother's voice and seems to sense things that will be ignored later. It is as if the baby is trying its best to win the affections of its parents.

The bonding which occurs soon after birth is said to be very important to the child's well-being as it grows up. Yet parents and children bond in different ways - some prefer less physical contact than others, for example. However, it is very important for every baby or child to know that he, or she, is loved and wanted by his, or her, parents.

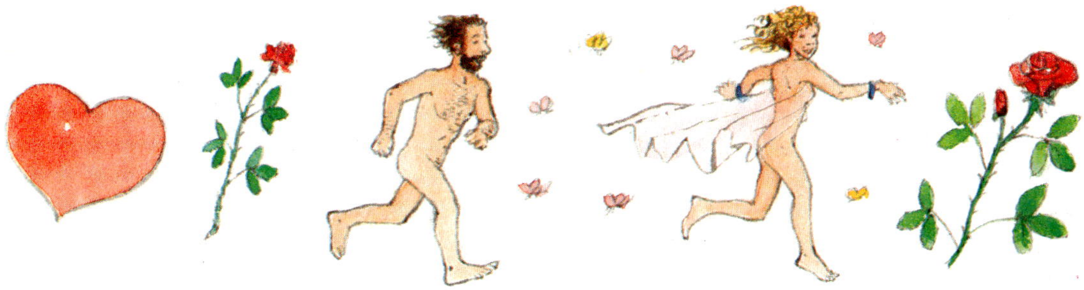

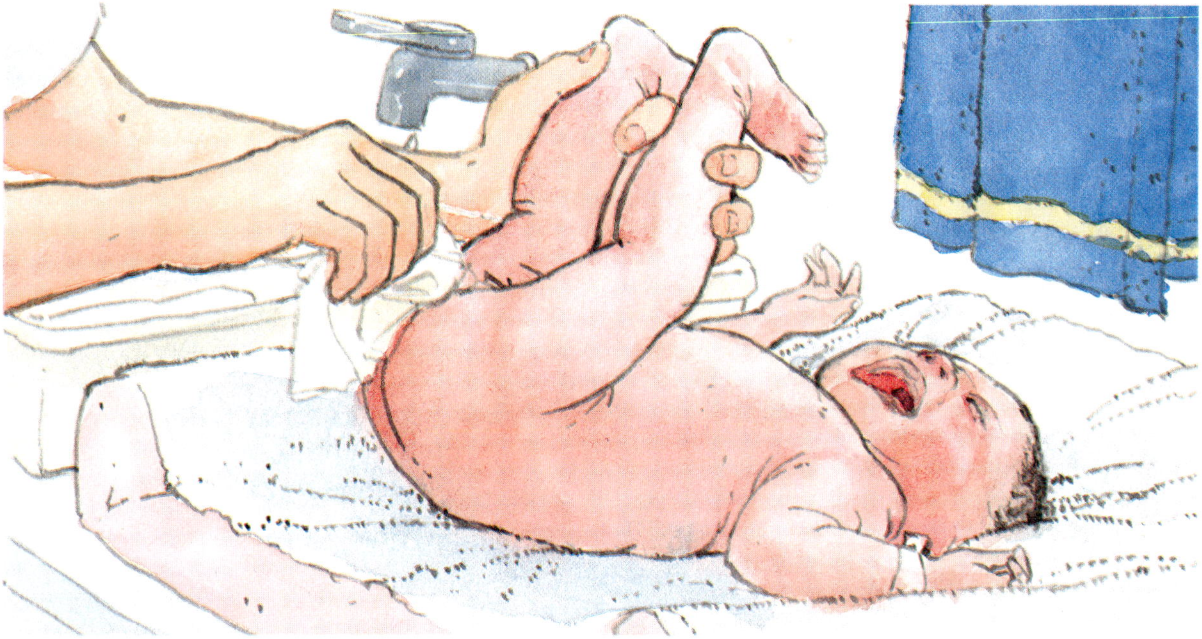

• What happens to the baby after birth?

Doctors or midwives always examine a newborn baby. He, or she, checks its breathing, its heart, its strength, its reflexes and the colour of its skin. If the baby is healthy, it is given to its mother.

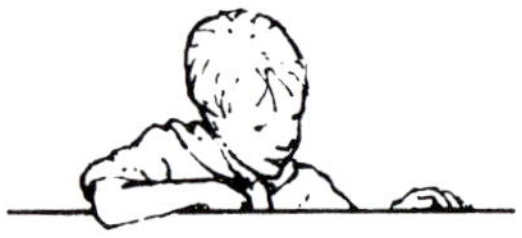

Auntie Karen told me that about five days after she had given birth to baby Sarah, the doctor had pricked one of Sarah's heels with a needle. He had taken the blood for tests to see if she had any diseases. Auntie Karen did not get the results of these tests, but the family doctor told her that everything was all right and that the hospital only released the results if there were any problems.

Robert, 11 years old

• What happens to the umbilical cord?

When the umibilical cord is cut and clamped off, the baby is left with a stump on its tummy. The stump must be kept dry and clean.
After seven to ten days the stump falls off. Nothing is left except a small scar on the navel. This soon heals and becomes known as the tummy button.

• What does the newborn infant eat?

During pregnancy, the mother's breasts will have swelled. Certain hormones will have stimulated the production of colostrum, a special kind of milk. When the newborn baby sucks at its mother's breasts, it is sucking colostrum. Colostrum is the best baby food. It is rich in some minerals and certain

vitamins, as well as containing plenty of proteins and carbohydrates. This special milk contains antibodies that protect the baby from infections.
Colostrum has less fat and sugar than normal baby milk so it is easier for the baby to digest.
True milk appears in the breasts three days after delivery. It is all the baby needs in the way of food and drink, and the flow of milk to the breast is stimulated by its sucking action.
The baby has to suck quite vigorously at the breast and in this way it develops its mouth and cheek muscles.
In addition, the baby enjoys cuddling up to its mother and this moment is important in creating a bond between mother and child.
Suckling has another advantage for the woman. When the baby suckles at the breast it causes the uterus to clamp down and reduce the flow of blood from where the placenta came away. The uterus returns to its normal shape faster if the woman breastfeeds. It also helps her to regain her figure.

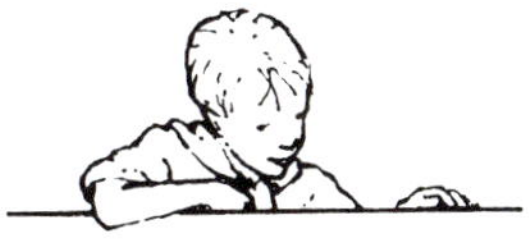

When my sister had a baby and she breastfed it, she was very careful about what she ate. She drank lots of water and avoided eating cabbages, peas, asparagus, onions and garlic. She cut down on strong curries and alcohol. She was careful not to eat too much fruit in case it would give her baby wind or indigestion.

Frank, 16 years old

Do small breasts produce less milk?

The size of breasts has nothing to do with the amount of milk they produce. Small breasts contain less fatty tissue. It is not the fatty tissue, but the glandular tissues of the mammary glands, that are important in producing milk.

• Do all mothers breastfeed?

Breastfeeding is generally considered to be beneficial for both mother and baby. Experts have proved that breastfeeding can reduce the risks of breast cancer.
Most women are able to breastfeed very well, but some may feel they have too little milk or that it would spoil the shape of their breasts.
Mothers who want to return to work soon after the baby is born cannot breastfeed during the day, while some mothers find that their nipples become too sore to continue breastfeeding.
Occasionally, if the woman is suffering from an illness which she risks passing on to her newborn infant through the milk, or if she is taking medications that would be harmful to it, the doctor will advise her not to breastfeed.
In such cases, the baby is given milk in a bottle. The milk is made from a powder which is added to boiled water. This milk is full of nutrients and it is almost as easy for the baby to digest as

The baby is losing weight...

During its first few days, the baby may lose a little weight. This weight loss is perfectly normal and it stops after about four or five days.

breast milk. Using a bottle to feed the baby has the added advantage that Daddy can help too.

• How does a mother know if her baby is drinking enough milk?

When a baby drinks milk from a bottle, the mother knows exactly how much it has drunk. Sucking milk from the breast is another matter and it is difficult to estimate how much milk a baby has taken in. This is why babies are weighed regularly every few days for the first couple of weeks. Provided that the baby's weight increases steadily, and the baby sleeps well (about six to eight hours a day), it can be assumed that it is drinking enough milk.

• How long are babies breastfed for?

It is up to the mother how long she wants to breastfeed for. Some mothers stop breastfeeding after a few weeks. Others continue until the baby is about one year old.

If it is breastfed, the baby needs no other form of food or drink until it is six months old. By then the baby is more active and the mother supplements its milk diet with baby rice or puréed fruit or vegetables. By the time a baby is about ten months old it may have started to eat minced or grated food.

• Is it possible to breastfeed twins?

Yes, it is perfectly possible to breastfeed twins. The more the breasts are sucked, the more milk is produced. It is usual for a mother to feed the twins separately, however, and take turns in feeding one before the other.

• What is post-natal depression?

When their baby has been born, most women are very happy. However, they can be very emotional at this time and even if they are happy to have had a baby, they may cry on and off during the first week after the birth. They may also feel depressed.
These feelings of sadness, which are sometimes called 'baby blues', are quite normal and not, in fact, anything to do with post-natal depression. This type of depression starts around the third or fourth week after delivery.
It is the result of changes to the hormonal balance and a woman who suffers from post-natal depression should see a doctor. She will need to be reassured by medical expertise that eventually the depression will lift.

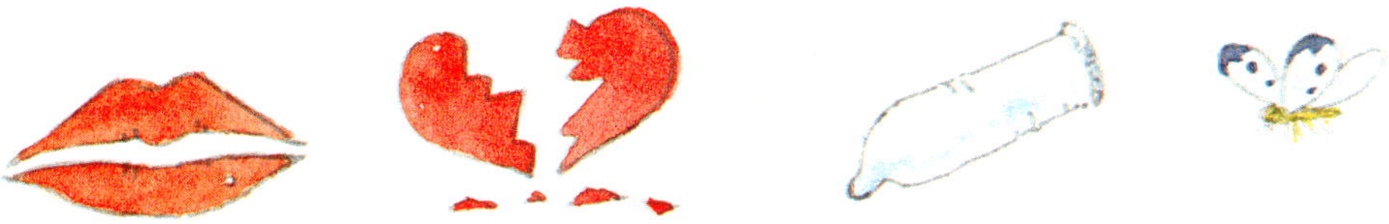
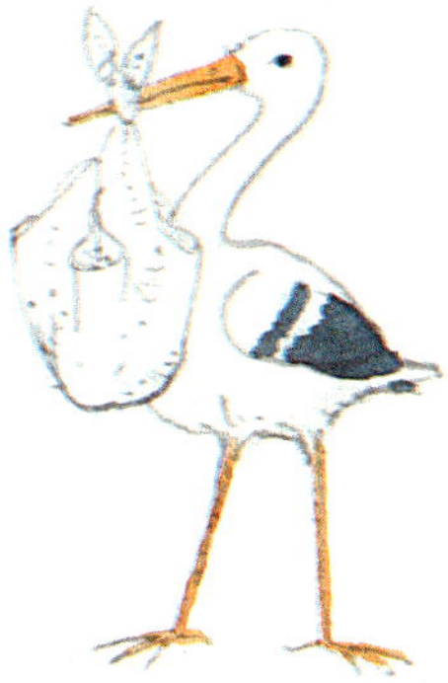

RELATIONSHIPS IN TODAY'S SOCIETY

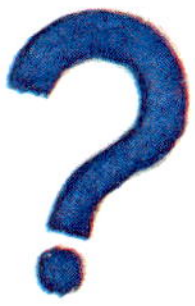

In the past, men and women were expected to get married and have children. Anything else was unacceptable and not talked about openly. Nowadays all sorts of relationships or sexual preferences are possible, but many of them are not clearly explained to adolescents. Consequently, teenagers develop odd ideas about such things as homosexuality or celibacy.
The following questions and answers aim to clear up any misconceptions about relationships in today's society. When children are approaching adulthood it is better that they know as much as possible so that they can be well prepared.

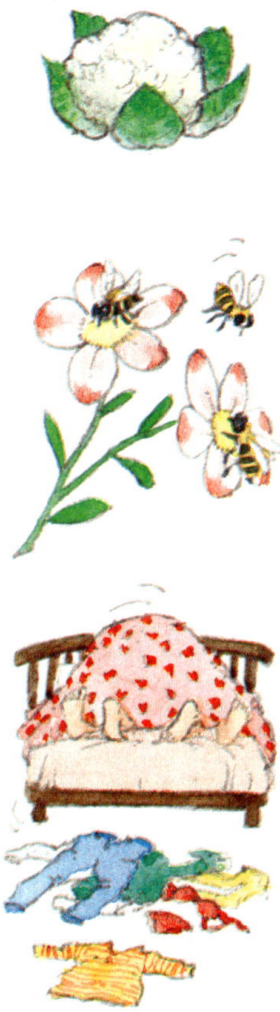

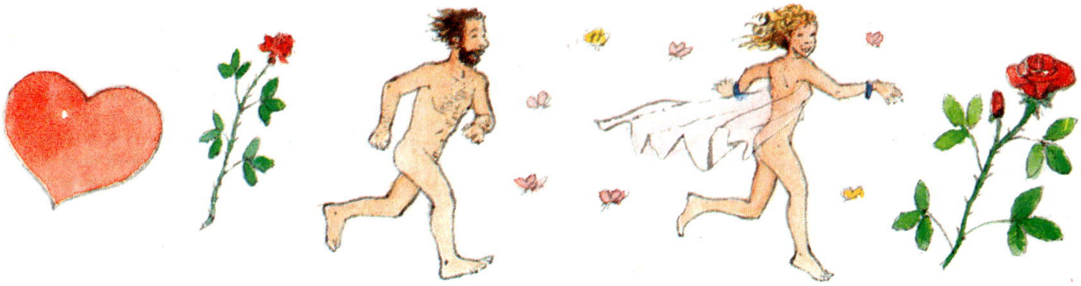

• What is a part-time relationship?

This is when a couple who are having a sexual relationship prefer to live apart. The man and woman each have their own flat or house and sometimes these are in different parts of the country. The couple live apart for most of the time, but they spend time together when the opportunity arises or when they both feel they want to. The idea of a part-time relationship is that each person keeps their own independence and respects the freedom of the other.

• What is a celibate mother?

A celibate mother is one who wants to have a child but who does not want to live with a man.

The woman looks for a man who is willing to make her pregnant and yet will not want to live with her or help with the child's upbringing.

This situation occasionally gives rise to all sorts of problems. For example, men who agreed to the idea in the first place, later want to stay in contact with the child or support it.

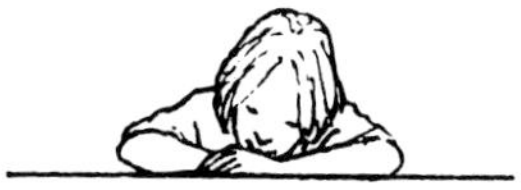

My brother is gay. He lives with his boyfriend in a house which they have bought together. They get on really well and I don't understand what people have got against homosexuals.

Frances, 15 years old

• What are homosexuals?

'Homo' and 'heteral' come from Greek words.

'Homo' means 'similar, the same' and 'heteros' means 'the other'. In other words, a homosexual is a man who has a sexual preference for another man, or a woman who has a sexual preference for another woman. A man who has a sexual preference for a woman (and vice versa) is heterosexual.

Homosexual women are often referred to as 'lesbians'. This word alludes to the ancient homosexual female poet, called Sapho, who lived on the Greek island of Lesbos.

Many homosexuals are ashamed of their homosexuality because society has encouraged an unfavourable opinion of them. Some are frightened of being excluded from society or of losing their jobs, or even of being attacked.

This is sad because they cannot help their sexual preference and they are not guilty of any crime.

During adolescence, teenagers may discover that they are different from their friends. For example, a girl may fall in love with another girl or a boy may be attracted to another boy. This attraction disturbs and frightens them and often they dare not talk about their feelings to anyone, not even to their parents. It is common, however, for adolescents to feel attracted to people of the same sex without actually becoming homosexual.

It is usually just a passing phase in their development and they grow out of it when they fall in love with someone of the opposite sex.

• What is prostitution?

It is said that prostitution is the oldest profession in the world. Prostitutes are women (or in certain cases, men) who have sex in return for money. They work in massage parlours or pick up customers on the streets of red light areas. Some prostitutes choose their occupation by preference, others are forced into it against their will. Many have had an unhappy childhood and come from broken homes or they have fallen on hard times.

Most prostitutes work for pimps. These are men who control the red light districts where prostitutes normally work. Pimps take a large proportion of the money that the women have earned, often against their will. In return, the pimps provide customers, as well as some protection from people who want to cause the prostitutes harm.

Unfortunately, pimps sometimes bully and hurt the women to make them earn more money. They may also force them to perform unnatural sexual acts for certain customers.

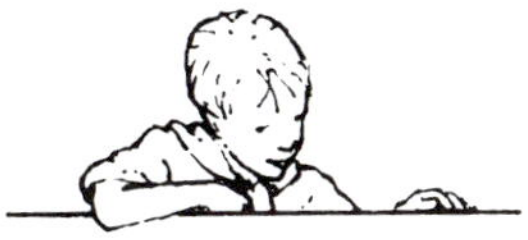

When I come back from school, I walk down a road where there are some prostitutes waiting for customers. They wear very short skirts and high heels. Sometimes they try to attract my attention, but I ignore them. My father has told me what they are doing and I think it sounds weird.

Steven, 12 years old

• What is rape?

Rape means forcing someone to have sexual intercourse against their will. Rape can be committed by a stranger, a friend, or even within marriage.

Some men refuse to listen to women when they say they do not want to have sex.

They continue making sexual advances and this leads to rape.

Rape is an act of violence that is very upsetting for the victim. It is a serious criminal offence.

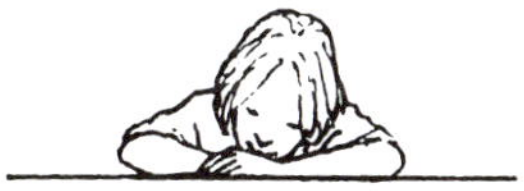

My father read in a newspaper about a sadist who raped and beat a girl of 14 to death. My father was very upset about it because I am 14 too. He said he hoped the sadist would spend the rest of his life in prison.

Barbara, 14 years old

Tricked!

Sometimes Asian women are tricked into going to Western countries with the promise of a job.

When they arrive, however, the women find they are forced to work as prostitutes in order to earn enough money to repay the airfare and for their upkeep.

• What are sexual deviations?

Normal sexual behaviour is not enough for some people, who develop unusual sexual preferences. This includes exhibitionism, sadism and masochism.
Below are brief descriptions of some of the more common deviations, otherwise referred to as sexual perversions.

Voyeurism
Voyeurism derives from the French word 'voyer' meaning 'to see', or 'to look'. A voyeur is someone who enjoys secretly watching people getting undressed or when they are naked. In most cases, voyeurs do not cause any harm, but it is an arrestable offence.

Exhibitionism
An exhibitionist is a man who takes pleasure in exposing his private parts in public. Such a person will stop a girl or woman in a park or street and show her his penis.
It is an alarming experience for any woman but generally these men are not dangerous.

Transvestitism
A transvestite is a man who gets sexually excited by dressing up in woman's clothes. He puts on make-up, a wig and copies the way a woman walks and moves.

Masochism
A masochist is someone who can only get sexual pleasure by being physically hurt or mentally humiliated.
In very extreme cases this behaviour may prove fatal.

Sadism
A sadist enjoys inflicting pain on someone else. This may range from gentle punishment, such as a slap, to an unacceptable level of violence. Sadism may involve pretending to be a person in authority who dominates the victim for sexual pleasure.

Paedophilia
Paedophilia is when a man forces a child to have sex with him. Children are not physically ready for sex and it is a serious criminal offence for a man to have sexual intercourse with anyone under the age of 16.
Paedophilia is extremely distressing for the child, who is mentally and physically damaged by it.

THE QUESTIONS IN THIS BOOK

• In what ways are boys and girls different?

• Fertilisation

• Making love

• From embryo to baby

• Birth

INDEX

This edition by: Invader, England.
Illustrations: K. Nauwelaerts.
Printed in Belgium.